Managing Tic and Habit Disorders

Managing Tic and Habit Disorders

A Cognitive Psychophysiological Approach
with Acceptance Strategies

Kieron P. O'Connor

Marc E. Lavoie

Benjamin Schoendorff

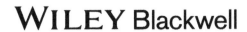

Registered Office(s)
John Wiley & Sons, Inc., 111 River Street, Hoboken, NJ 07030, USA
John Wiley & Sons Ltd, The Atrium, Southern Gate, Chichester, West Sussex, PO19 8SQ, UK

Editorial Office
The Atrium, Southern Gate, Chichester, West Sussex, PO19 8SQ, UK

For details of our global editorial offices, customer services, and more information about Wiley products visit us at www.wiley.com.

Wiley also publishes its books in a variety of electronic formats and by print-on-demand. Some content that appears in standard print versions of this book may not be available in other formats.

Library of Congress Cataloging-in-Publication Data Is Available
9781119167259 [hardback]
9781119167273 [paperback]
9781119167297 [ePDF]
9781119167280 [ePub]

Cover image: © Zoonar RF/Gettyimages
Cover design: Wiley

Set in 10/12pt Warnock Pro by SPi Global, Pondicherry, India

10 9 8 7 6 5 4 3 2 1

Contents

List of Tables and Figures

Tables

Figures

About the Authors

Kieron P. O'Connor obtained his doctorate from the Institute of Psychiatry in London. He is currently Director of the Obsessive-Compulsive Disorder and Tic Disorder Studies Centre at the University Institute of Mental Health at Montreal, and Centre Integré Universitaire de Santé et de Service Sociaux de L'Est de l'Ile de Montréal; Full Professor at the Psychiatry Department of University of Montréal; and Associated Professor at the University of Quebec. He is a Fellow of the Canadian Psychology Association and Associate Fellow of the British Psychological Society. His interests include treatment of obsessive-compulsive disorders, eating disorders, dissociative disorders, delusional disorders, and tic and body focused repetitive disorders. He directs a clinical research program currently funded by the Canadian Institutes of Health Research and the Quebec Health Research fund aimed at studying the interaction of cognitive, psycho-physiological, psychosocial, and behavioral factors in the management of psychological problems. He is author or co-author of over 200 scientific articles, reports, and books, and frequently leads formations and workshops on innovative approaches to treating belief disorders.

Marc E. Lavoie investigates the link between cognitive processes and cerebral activity (event-related potentials), primarily in Tourette's syndrome. He works closely with psychological intervention teams to identify psychophysiological changes that occur following cognitive-behavioral therapy. He is a Professor of Psychiatry and Neuroscience at the University of Montréal, and is currently Head of the Cognitive and Social Psychophysiology Laboratory, at the research center of the Institut Universitaire en Santé Mentale de Montréal, which addresses crucial issues about the relationship between brain functions, behavior, and cognition in various neuropsychiatric disorders.

Benjamin Schoendorff, MA, MSc, is a clinical psychologist and Director of the Contextual Psychology Institute in Montréal, Canada. A renowned international acceptance and commitment therapy (ACT) trainer, he has authored and co-authored several ACT books in French and English. He has co-edited *The ACT Matrix* (2014), and co-authored *The ACT Practitioner's Guide to the Science of Compassion* (2014) and, most recently, *The Essential Guide to the ACT Matrix* (2016). He loves traveling with his wife and young son Thomas. www.contextpsy.com.

Acknowledgments

The authors would like to thank the therapists who have applied the therapy in practice: Natalia Koszegi, Genevieve Goulet, Veronica Muschang, Genevieve Paradis, Vicky Leblanc, Jeremy Dohan, Vicky Auclair, and Danielle Gareau.

The following people contributed substantially to the realization of the book: Karine Bergeron, Annette Maillet, Nick Delarosbil-Huard, Julie Leclerc, and Catherine Courchesne. Yuliya and Victoria Bodryzlova helped with the indexing.

We would like to thank the production team at Wiley-Blackwell.

Finally, we would like to thank our clients who took part in the study, who inspired our treatment and permitted the experimental validation of our model.

About the Companion Website

The electronic supplemental content to support the use of this text is available online at www.wiley.com/go/oconnor/managingticandhabitdsorders

Introduction

Kieron P. O'Connor, Marc E. Lavoie, and Benjamin Schoendorff

Cognitive-behavioral management complements the neurodevelopmental aspects of tic and habit disorders. In the chapters that follow, we describe a new and improved therapist and accompanying client manual of our tic and habit management program: the cognitive psychophysiological approach (CoPs) (O'Connor, 2005). The program has widened to include psychosocial, metacognitive, and other behavioral aspects, which we combine with acceptance strategies. We have now carried out over 20 years of clinical research dealing with tics or habits, during which time we have conducted a number of clinical trials and neuropsychological work. Our research has informed our opinion that tics or habits are really the tip of the iceberg; that there are background behavioral aspects influencing tics or habits; that tics or habits are embedded in personal activity; that surrounding psychosocial and thought processes define tics or habits; and that tics or habits interact with how we perceive others and our own activities. So, although tics or habits may well serve a short-term function in reducing stress, so producing reinforcing consequences that immediately maintain them, they are also products of a context of cognitive-behavioral psychophysiological activity occurring prior to and during their occurrence (see Figure 0.1).

The program has been validated for both tic and habit disorders (the user friendly term we use for bodily focused repetitive behaviors, BFRBs) so the manual addresses both disorders, which, despite some differences, we consider to be part of the same spectrum of disorders. Tic or habit onset may be an inevitable endpoint of tension built up as a result of the way action is planned and executed. So the tic or habit, often arising locally, is not the focus here—in fact we recommend accepting the tic or habit when it occurs, rather than fighting the tic or habit or holding it in, contracting or disguising it: all self-sabotaging strategies that tend to exacerbate the underlying tension. Rather, we encourage developing a flow of action and moving past the tic or habit toward goals, and heading smoothly and effortlessly toward goal-directed planning activity.

The CoPs model is a comprehensive model taking into account, as the name implies, cognitive, physiological, and emotional dimensions, and treating the client holistically. It is predicated on two sound assertions:

1) That thinking and physiology are interlinked. This is not obvious since clients have often considered the tic or habit problem as purely neurological. But tics

Managing Tic and Habit Disorders: A Cognitive Psychophysiological Approach with Acceptance Strategies, First Edition. Kieron P O'Connor, Marc E Lavoie, and Benjamin Schoendorff.
© 2017 John Wiley & Sons, Ltd. Published 2017 by John Wiley & Sons, Ltd.
Companion Website: www.wiley.com/go/oconnor/managingticandhabitdsorders

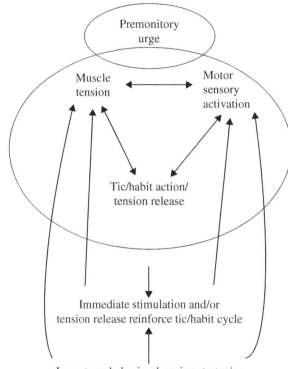

Figure 0.1 Local immediate triggers and reinforcing tic or habit cycle

or habits are best viewed as psychophysiological, which is to say that the physiological elements of ticking are often modulated by psychological factors, which include: behavior, mood, social setting, and perceived external triggers. The effects are two-way, and change in behavior can influence change in physiology. In particular, thought processes involved in anticipation and preparation can be triggers for ticking and are a key connection between thoughts and physiology.

2) There is an important distinction between controlling the tic or habit and achieving a sense of mastery from being able to prevent the tic or habit through mastery over the processes that build up to it. We make the distinction between positive acceptance and mastery, and a negative fighting and containing type of control over the tic or habit.

The cognitive element is also essential to the program in the sense that we encourage exercises to enhance awareness or, as we choose to call it, discovery. In fact awareness is about discovery and bringing new elements into consciousness, but discovery is also actively exploring and integrating new knowledge about the nature of the client's tic or habit, like exploring a new land, sailing down the stream along a new river—a metaphor that fits well within the steps of the program (see client manual).

This manual addresses both tics and what we call habit disorders (the technical name is bodyfocused repetitive behaviors), including hair pulling, nail biting, skin picking, and skin scratching. These problems are distinct and vary on several dimensions, but they seem to respond to the same treatment, namely CoPs, and share features in common. Although BFRBs or habits may require additional strategies, particularly regarding emotional regulation, we decided to deal with tics and habits together since they fall under the same tic or habit-like spectrum, despite differences in awareness and action motivating people, and clinicians often ask: is the problem a tic or a habit disorder?

We provide guidelines to distinguish tics and habits and other movement disorders. But we do suggest that the client consult a medical professional such as a neurologist to receive a diagnosis.

A Cognitive-Behavioral Psychophysiological Model of Tension Buildup

So what are the ingredients of the CoPs model of tic or habit onset and maintenance? The CoPs model integrates physiological and behavioral aspects as well as cognitive and emotional experiences. It paints a comprehensive picture of the interactions between the physiological dimensions of muscle tension, ticking, and behavior, and cognitive and emotional patterns that may feed tics and habit disorders. The key theme of the program is developing flexibility in muscles, planning, thinking, emotional coping, self-talk, and self-judgment. On the psychophysiological side, heightened sensory awareness, an overactive behavioral style, and impulsive tendencies contribute to the onset and maintenance of tics or habits, while, on the cognitive side, perfectionism regarding self-image, personal standards, and a dysfunctional way of approaching planning of action are implicated. People with tics or habits often display somewhat perfectionist beliefs about the importance of being efficient, doing as much as possible, and not wasting time or appearing to do so. On the action side, they attempt too much at once, have trouble pacing action, invest more effort than necessary in a given task, and abandon tasks prematurely. They are also unwilling to relax, have trouble being present in the here and now, and tend to overinvest in trying to foresee the unforeseeable. Finally, rather than using visual feedback of a particular action, people with tics or habits may pay more heed to more general proprioceptive information, leading them to tense until they attain a sense of "feeling just right," or have felt they put the right amount of effort into a task. In fact, tics and habits may be providing just such a muscle focused feedback by occupying the client in a proprioceptive loop, which gives the impression of "doing something" in situations where normal goal directed activity is frustrated. Also people with habit disorders in particular, but also some people with tics or habits, experience a lot of self-criticism and shame about themselves, and generally find it difficult to cope with negative emotions, which can trigger the habit (see Figures 0.2 and 0.3). So we suggest that more compassionate ways of viewing the self and accepting self and emotions may help with control.

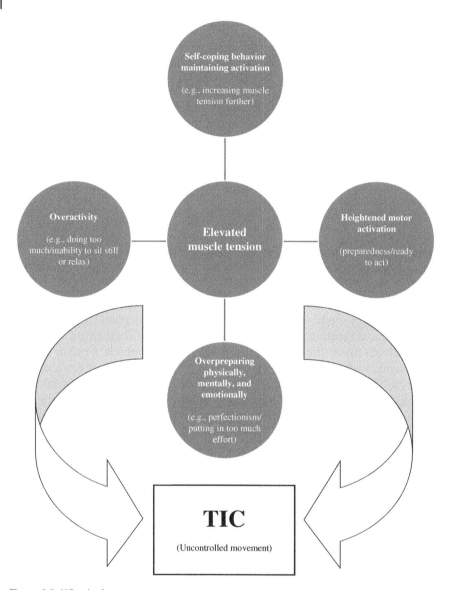

Figure 0.2 Why tics happen

Structure of the Program

In line with our model, the *first* part of the program describes the history of Tourette's, tic disorders, and habit disorders, current thinking on etiology, and the growing recognition of the utility of behavioral interventions. The *second* part considers all aspects, both psychosocial and clinical, needed for a comprehensive diagnostic and psychological assessment. The formal semi-structured interviews are cited but not explored; rather, focus is on evaluations essential to

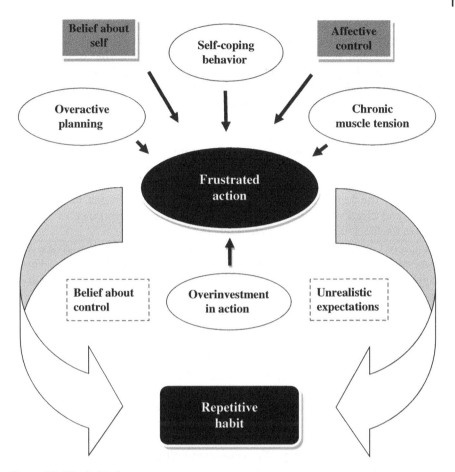

Figure 0.3 Why habits happen

the program. Included in evaluation is a look at how the client and other people judge the problem, and the problem of stigma and living with and communicating about the problem. The *third* section involves steps of the program, beginning with motivation and education about the close link between thoughts and actions and the way that sometimes how we react to our tics and habits leads to self-sabotaging strategies. We discuss discovery and awareness exercises to help the client learn about the nature and form of their tic or habit. The role of tension in triggering the tic or habit in action is illustrated, along with exercises to improve muscle flexibility, discrimination between muscles, and relaxation. High and low risk activities/situations for tic onset are evaluated, and how these reveal existing strengths and control and also give us an insight into how evaluations can influence tensions. The importance of obtaining cognitive and physical flexibility is highlighted, with exercises to improve flexibility and efficient muscle use, and showing how to focus on acceptance of the tic or habit whilst avoiding strategies that lead the client away from goals. Rethinking the client's entire style of planning in order to prevent tic or habit onset by using existing strengths in the client's repertoire and planning less effortful action is encouraged, as well as improving emotional regulation and self-perception, particularly in body focused disorders or habit disorders. We also cover the important role of the B.e.s.t. Buddy and social support, and inform on how to ensure such feedback is helpful. Finally, we provide guidelines on maintaining gains by generalizing control through reference to the program and adopting future lifestyle changes to reinforce the client's new non-tic or non-habit life, and better identify and realize the client's goals and values. Each chapter discusses a separate module relevant to the program, but the chapters are planned as cumulative and progress logically.

The book is accompanied by a client manual containing steps and exercises, and designed and structured to accompany the main therapist manual. Throughout the therapist and client manuals we provide exercises, forms, information, and checks on motivation, and emphasize the importance of various forms of feedback in maintaining confidence.

Chapters 1 and 2 cover information on tics and habits, and how to assess and differentiate the two disorders from each other and non-clinical problems. These chapters are essential parts of the program and provide the knowledge required to progress further.

The third chapter addresses: motivation and goals of seeking treatment; how to maintain confidence throughout the program; surmounting obstacles; entertaining realistic expectations about the end result of the process; and, in particular, maintaining confidence through feedback from others following the program, rewards, changing one's perception of and talking differently about the tic or habit, and understanding the process of control.

Chapter 4 describes the important process of choosing and describing a principal tic or habit. We need to know what it looks like, the muscles implicated, and background activities. The discovery of the tic or habit can involve the B.e.s.t. Buddy, video, or diary. We recommend all three, and particularly the diary, which measures control, intensity, and frequency of tics or habits each day of the program, and gives an idea of progress. In keeping the diary, the client also discovers variations in tic or habit parameters that we systematize later. In monitoring, the client also becomes aware of upstream process preceding the buildup of tension and downstream processes occurring at the same time: as the tic or habit.

In Chapter 5, we systematize the variation in terms of high and low risk activities, in which the tic or habit is likely or unlikely to appear, and then find out how these evaluated differently, and what distinguishes the way the client thinks about high and low risk situations. We show how their anticipation of activities links to different types of often rigid beliefs about how to act.

We provide exercises and examples. We also expand our model, explaining how the principal aim is to address cognitive-behavioral and physiological processes preceding tension buildup and tic or habit onset, and introducing more flexibility into these processes.

In Chapter 6 we move onto consider flexibility in muscles and how the tension before ticking is often the result of conflicting preparation and unhelpful attempts at self-management. In line with the previous discussion of flow, we suggest adopting mindfulness, rather than conflict.

In Chapter 7, we continue the quest for flexibility in discrimination exercises, where we discuss the important of developing awareness of tension cues, particularly in the tic or habit affected muscles, and also employing unnecessary affect, particularly where the affect may be a criterion for performance. We move into relaxation in the whole body and the acceptance of sensations rather than fighting them or reacting to them.

In Chapter 8, we address the importance of being flexible in planning: planning in people with tics and habits often involves thinking and acting in an effortful way and investing too much. We discuss the behavioral cost of these tension-producing strategies and also how often these styles of planning action, typical of high risk situations, are driven by perfectionist thoughts. We then look at how we can plan to do less and be more flexible in planning to do less.

In Chapter 9 we explore how being more flexible can help the client approach rather than avoid their goals, and how often in thinking we may mix up figurative speech with reality: often what seems to be rigid thinking maybe simply taking literally an emotive statement and taking thoughts as reality, or taking them too seriously because we are used to them, rather than moving on. The matrix helps distinguish thoughts from reality in planning style of action.

Chapter 10 focuses on the importance of emotional investment in habits. Habits not only release tension, but form an emotional regulation often due to triggers involving self-judgment, self-criticism, and shame. It is important to validate emotions, but not necessarily act on them; to treat them as thoughts. Working with self-talk can help here, since it is important for the client to speak to him or herself compassionately—we can become hooked on words and their meanings, taking them more seriously than we should.

Finally, in Chapter 11, we discuss maintaining the gains the client has made by continuing to practice, revision of the new program, selective application of the program to new tics and habits, changing other aspects of the client's lifestyle, and continuing with social support and positive feedback, compassion and rewards, and a recognition of the client's accomplishments.

The companion client manual can be downloaded and follows closely the structure of the program laid out in the therapist manual but addressed from a client's point of view.

1

The Nature of Tics and Habits

Overview of the Nature of Tics and Habits

History

The first references to tics go back to medieval times. In the fifteenth century, two Dominican monks reported the case of a priest who could not help but grimace and emit vocalizations, whenever he was praying (Kramer and Sprenger, 1948). Later in 1825, Jean-Marc Gaspard Itard described tics in a systematic way for the first time (Itard, 1825). The latter reports the case of a 26-year-old French noblewoman, the Marquise de Dampierre, who presented involuntary convulsive spasms and contortions at the level of the shoulders, neck, and face. Shortly afterwards, he also reported the presence of "spasms affecting the organs of voice and speech," and notes the presence of strange screams and senseless words in the absence of a circumscribed mental disorder.

The Gilles de la Tourette syndrome is named after the French neurologist Georges Gilles de la Tourette, who, in 1885, described again the condition of the Marquise de Dampierre, now aged 86 years old, who continued to make abrupt movements and sounds also known as tics. The same year, Tourette described eight other patients with motor and vocal tics, some of whom had echo phenomena (a tendency to repeat things said to them) and coprolalia (utterances of obscene phrases) (Gilles de la Tourette, 1885) which was consistent with similar observations from American clinicians 1 year later (see Dana & Wilkin, 1886). In a doctoral dissertation published under the supervision of Tourette and Charcot, Jacques Catrou, documented 26 other cases (Catrou, 1890) with more details. The merit of Gilles de la Tourette's report, consisted not only in gathering remarkable clinical descriptions of the symptoms that were little documented, if ever, until then, but also in describing the fluctuating evolution of what become known as the Gilles de la Tourette Syndrome (Gilles de la Tourette, 1885).

Subsequently, there were few systematic investigations, clinical observations, or particular etiological developments during the first half of the twentieth century. Rather, during this period, a psychoanalytic explanation prevailed, with little or no notable empirical support (Ascher, 1948; Ferenczi, 1921; Mahler, 1944; Mahler, Luke, & Daltroff, 1945). In the 1960s an experimental drug treatment (i.e., haloperidol) surfaced for tics (Seignot, 1961). These results encouraged clinical trials in the United States, which further supported the beneficial effects of neuroleptics (Corbett, Mathews, Connell, & Shapiro, 1969; Shapiro 1970; Shapiro & Shapiro, 1968). These seminal investigations instigated the race to find an effective pharmacological treatment and, therefore, the search for a neurobiological etiology, relegating to the background, the psychoanalytic, and the behavioral approach as well (Shapiro & Shapiro, 1971 Shapiro, 1970; 1976).

Idea of a Tourette or Tic and Habit Spectrum

A majority of patients with Tourette's also face various concomitant problems (Freeman et al., 2000), which include obsessive-compulsive disorder (OCD) or at least some obsessive-compulsive symptoms, attention deficit hyperactivity disorder (ADHD), depression, and anxiety disorders.

Current Diagnostic Criteria of Tics and Habits

Nosology of the Gilles de la Tourette syndrome and tic disorders

Tic disorder and Tourette's syndrome are currently classified in the Diagnostic and Statistical Manual of Mental Disorders Version 5 (DSM-5) (APA, 2013) with motor disorders listed in the neurodevelopmental disorder category. A tic is defined as a sudden, rapid, recurrent, non-rhythmic motor movement or vocalization. Tics can be present in the form of simple or complex multiple motor or vocal tics. The complex tics are contractions of a group of skeletal muscles, resulting in complex and repetitive movements, such as hopping, contact with certain objects or people, grimacing, abdominal spasms, tapping, movements or extension of the arms or legs, shoulder movements in sequence, copropraxia (unintentionally performing sexual gestures), or echokinesia (imitation of a gesture). Simple tics are defined as non-voluntary repetitive contractions of functionally related groups of skeletal muscles in one or more parts of the body including blinking, cheek twitches, and head jerks among others. Vocal tics can also take the form of simple (e.g., coughing, sniffing, clearing throat) or complex tics, such as coprolalia (using profanity and obscene words) or palilalia (involuntary repetition of syllables, words, or phrases).

Tic disorders are grouped into three main classifications in the DSM-5: Tourette's disorder (307.23), persistent chronic motor or vocal tic disorder (307.22), and provisional tic disorder (307.21).

The criteria for Tourette's disorder are (a) the presence of both multiple motor and one or more vocal tics at some time during the illness, although not necessarily concurrently; (b) tics that may wax and wane in frequency, but have persisted for more than 1 year since first onset; (c) onset is before age 18 years; and (d) a disturbance that is not attributable to the physiological effects of a substance or another medical condition (e.g., Huntington's disease, post-viral encephalitis). For the persistent chronic motor or vocal tic disorder, single or

Table 1.1 Examples of simple and complex tics

Parts of body	Involuntary repetitive movements
Mental	Playing a tune or phrase over and over in your head, mentally counting numbers for no apparent reason. Following contours with the eyes or in the mind
Head	Head tics to the side, front, or back. Tapping or hitting the head
Face	Nose wrinkling, ear flapping, cheek contracting, forehead and temple tension, raising eyebrows, licking or biting lips, protruding tongue
Eyes	Winking, excessive blinking, eyelid tremor, squinting, straining eye muscles, staring, rolling eyes, opening eyes excessively
Mouth	Lip movement, chewing, teeth grinding, tongue ducking, parsing, pouting, forcing tongue against palate, biting tongue, biting finger nails
Vocal/phonic	Coughing, burping, throat clearing, humming, making noises, swallowing, repeating phrases or tunes, sniffing, laughing, breathing, swearing
Shoulders	Movement shrug up and down or forwards or backwards or on one side
Abdomen	Tensing stomach or abdomen into a knot, expanding the abdomen
Torso	Tensing, twisting, or gyrating movement involving legs, arms, or trunk. Maintaining a fixed posture
Hands	Rubbing fingers together, waggling or clinching fingers or cracking fingers or knuckles, scratching, twiddling, doodling, tapping, fidgeting, stroking (earlobes, chin, etc.), playing with objects, clenching/unclenching the fist.
Legs	Moving legs repetitively up and down or towards and away from each other, bending legs, kicking movements

Note: *Cognitive or mental tics* are controversial, but involve mental repetitions of words/phrases/tunes/maneuvers that are mostly not visible but respond in the same way to the program. Often they can be substituted for motor tics, which become equally uncontrollable and distressing. They have a situational profile and are accompanied by specific motor actions, eye movements, postures, behavior, and similar processes preceding onset. It is important to distinguish mental tics from obsessions, which are anxiogenic. Mental tics are frequently playful and stimulating at the beginning, but can later become invasive but are unrelated to a dominant fear. Similarly, *sensory tics* generally involve some tension associated with the sensation, such as tingling, burning, or itching, and may be independent phenomena or a precursor or consequence of behavior to follow.

multiple motor or vocal tics have been present during the illness, but not both motor and vocal. The other criteria are similar to those for Tourette's disorder.

In provisional tic disorder single or multiple motor and/or vocal tics are present, and tics have been present for less than 1 year since first tic onset. Criteria have never been met for Tourette's disorder or persistent (chronic) motor or vocal tic disorder (see examples in Table 1.1).

Habit disorders and body focused repetitive behavior (BFRB)

Another concomitant clinical problem often associated with tic disorder is body focused repetitive behavior (BFRB), also known as habit disorder. BFRB represents a clinical term that includes various diagnoses, such as trichotillomania,

Table 1.2 Examples of body focused repetitive disorder of hair pulling, skin picking, nail biting, neck cracking, body symmetry, and idiosyncratic

Hair pulling	Skin picking	Nail biting
• Recurrent pulling out of own hair, resulting in noticeable hair loss • Hair may also be eaten or rolled into balls and swallowed	• Repetitive picking of blemishes or healthy skin causing tissue damage using fingers, tweezers, pins, or other instruments	• Insertion of fingers into mouth, with contact between nails and teeth • Teeth replace scissors or nail clippers • Nail often bitten beyond nail bed and cuticles, drawing blood
Neck cracking	**Body symmetry**	**Idiosyncratic**
• Twitching neck or flexing knuckles until joints crack and crack is felt or heard	• Complex body movements to even up feeling of symmetry on either side	• Any self-destructive repetitive movements to give feeling of relief and emotional regulation

skin picking, and onychophagia, and may also include certain types of teeth grinding. More precisely, habits are impulsive and destructive body focused behaviors that are repetitive, automatic, and serve no obvious function. These include hair pulling (trichotillomania; TTM), skin picking (BS), nail biting (NB), teeth grinding, and knuckle cracking, among others. They are variably described as impulse control disorder, stereotypic movement disorder, and obsessive-compulsive spectrum disorders (see definitions of each habit disorder in Table 1.2).

Despite the heterogeneity of symptoms in the BFRB category, their main clinical signs are directed toward the body, in reaction to feelings of discomfort, which is often present in tic disorder. In the Diagnostic and Statistical Manual of Mental Disorders, Fourth Edition, text revision (DSM-IV-TR), trichotillomania was categorized as an impulse control disorder, not elsewhere classified, and was associated with skin picking and onychophagia (APA, 2000). In the DSM-5, trichotillomania and skin picking are now classified within the obsessive-compulsive and related disorders category, while onychophagia and dermatophagia are mentioned as "other specified obsessive-compulsive and related disorders." According to the current diagnostic criteria, typically patients must have BFRB when they repeatedly engage in body focused activities (other than hair pulling or skin picking), make repeated attempts to reduce or stop the behaviors, and experience significant distress or impairment caused by the behaviors. Despite the fact that these disorders have been relocated to the obsessive-compulsive category, impulse control and feeling of sensory discomfort remain an important communality of their profile. In addition, this incapacity to resist a specific impulse or urge is a characteristic shared by tic disorder and BFRB patients.

Tic disorder and BFRB or habit disorders are considered similar, and the relationship between these two entities is sometimes clinically unclear: the complex movements in BFRB can often be confused with complex tics. Another good

Table 1.3 Impact of habits and physical and psychological sequelae

Physical	Psychological
• Hair loss, follicle damage, scalp irritation, repetitive strain injuries • Skin scarring, sores, and infections • Damage to fingers, gums, and teeth • Joint dislocation	• Shame, guilt, and embarrassment • Avoidance of swimming, windy weather, visiting hairdresser, doctor, and dentist • Significant social and occupational impairment

reason to characterize tic disorder and BFRB together is mainly related to their response to treatment. Our experience allows us to see habits as part of the Tourette spectrum. Table 1.3 gives a list of all problem habits that we consider to fall under the Tourette/tic/habit spectrum and why. We do not include bruxism (teeth grinding), although it responds well to the CoPs treatment program.

Current Multidimensional Etiology of Tics and Habits

Prevalence, comorbidity, and behavioral problems

Once considered an uncommon syndrome, the Gilles de la Tourette Syndrome is no longer considered as a rare condition and is now regarded as being almost as common as schizophrenia. The DSM-IV-TR set the current prevalence rate of 5 to 30 children out of 10 000 and 1 to 2 adults out of 10 000 (APA, 2000). The Tourette International Consortium reported that the male to female ratio is 4.4 to 1 with a mean age of onset of 6.4 years (Freeman, 2007). A family history is present in 52% of patients, while attention deficit hyperactivity disorder (ADHD) is observed in 56%, and obsessive compulsive disorder (OCD) is observed in 55%. In terms of clinical course, tics tend to disappear in adult life in approximately half of patients and remain in only 10% of patients (Robertson et al., 2012). However, some authors claim that this proportion is inaccurate due to the variance characterizing the target population (Lanzi et al., 2004; Leclerc, Forget, & O'Connor, 2008). Current epidemiological studies indicate a prevalence of 1 individual in 200 would be more realistic, especially due to the presence of comorbid disorders (Freeman et al., 2000; Hornsey, Banerjee, Zeitlin, & Robertson, 2001; Kadesjö & Gillberg, 2000; Mason, Banerjee, Eapen, Zeitlin, & Robertson, 1998; Wang & Kuo, 2003). Furthermore, as noted by O'Connor (2005), the presence of tics or habits may be an important source of distress. This can take the form of phobias, depression, social anxiety, concerns about self-image, a decrease in self-esteem, relationship problems, and so on. The possible unsystematic presence of obscene gestures (copropraxia) or language (coprolalia) may also cause significant distress. In a study on the interference of tic disorder with daily activities, several socio-economic difficulties were reported: marital conflict, unemployment, mobility restrictions, and so on. This type of difficulty is perceived as being due to the presence of tics or

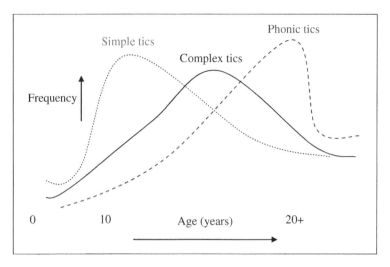

Figure 1.1 The development of tics

habits, but, to date, little epidemiological investigation has examined this field (O'Connor et al., 2001). Simple tics develop before complex tics and phonic tics (see Figure 1.1).

Neurological and physiological etiology

Understanding the cerebral causes of tic disorder remains important because it has the potential to help cognitive-behavioral therapy (CBT) practitioners to refine the modality according to motor symptoms as well as the corporeal distribution of tics or habits. This distribution, illustrated to the patient with a body diagram, helps to locate tics or habits during a structured interview. Tourette's syndrome has been considered initially to be of "nervous origin" even in the absence of an explanatory model of underlying symptoms (Gilles de la Tourette, 1885). Although important progress has been made in the past few decades due to, among other things, the series of seminal articles by the Shapiro team (Corbett, Matthews, Connell, & Shapiro, 1969; Shapiro, 1970, 1976; Shapiro & Shapiro, 1968), the cerebral origin of tics or habits remain, nonetheless, equivocal. Recent studies suggest that the mechanisms responsible for this syndrome could be attributed to a dopaminergic dysfunction provoking a higher level of cerebral activation than normal, so provoking these motor symptoms (Muller-Vahl et al., 2000). Dopamine is a neurotransmitter primarily associated with movement control as well as with rewards and pleasure. It is thus plausible to hypothesize that the networks associated with motor skills are involved in Tourette's syndrome. Neuroimaging studies have underlined the contribution of the frontal motor cortex as well as deeper subcortical regions such as the basal ganglia, which have been structurally affected among children and adults afflicted with Tourette's syndrome (Peterson et al., 2003). These deep nuclei project themselves via a structure called the thalamus and then to different

Neuroanatomy of tics

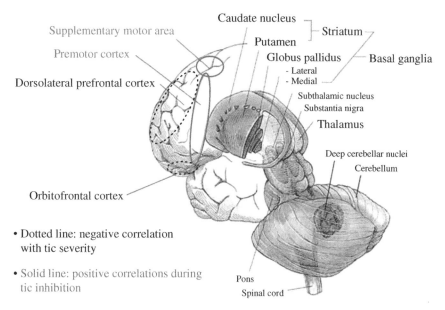

Figure 1.2 Illustration of the main regions affected in Tourette's syndrome Note: Obtained from magnetic resonance imaging, regions in dotted line were found to be negatively correlated with symptom severity, while the solid line areas are the regions that showed positive correlations with symptom severity. Moreover, before tic onset, significant activations were found in the region of the premotor cortex, while at tic onset sensorimotor and supplementary motor cortex activations were observed (Bohlhalter et al., 2006).

regions of the cortex also affected in Tourette's syndrome, such as the prefrontal and somatosensory cortex (Thomalla et al., 2009). These circuit loops are involved in multiple functions such as emotions, motivation, personality, disinhibition, executive functions, motor planning, and the control of different muscles. To date, this network is probably the best candidate for explaining the expression of tic symptoms (see Figure 1.2).

Somehow, the neurobiological hypothesis seems insufficient in order to truly appreciate the complexity of this syndrome, because we know little of the functional implication of affected structures in Tourette's syndrome. Is the entire network affected? Or is it a part of the network that affects other structures one after the other? Could it be an overactivation or an underactivation of certain networks?

Etiology of developmental and behavioral neuroplasticity in tics and habits

Tourette's syndrome is characterized by its fluctuating nature over time, and, as we have seen in the previous section, its developmental trajectory needs to be considered. Through longitudinal studies, certain hypotheses have underlined cerebral anomalies associated with the persistency of the symptoms in adulthood. Peterson and collaborators proposed that because it is present in every age group, certain brain alterations could constitute a global feature of Tourette's syndrome. However, the volume decrease of deep subcortical cerebral regions, as well as the increase in volume of cortical motor regions are uniquely present among adults, which suggests that they are associated with the development of symptom maintenance among subgroups with significant and persistent symptoms of Tourette's syndrome during adulthood. Among these individuals, there seems to be a neuroplasticity anomaly that allows counteracting for the presence of tics or habits via an overactivation of motor inhibition processes. Neuroplasticity is defined as the aptitude of the brain to alter its own structure and function following changes in the external environment, such as following a new learning concept or after psychotherapy, for instance. The brain could be able to adapt and realize such modifications following therapy, as demonstrated with neuroimaging (Deckersbach et al., 2014) and electrophysiological techniques (Lavoie, Imbriglio, Stip, & O'Connor, 2011; Morand-Beaulieu et al., 2016). According to that model, unlike adults, children with Tourette's syndrome have a relatively larger orbitofrontal volume (Peterson, 2001; Peterson et al., 2001; Spessot, Plessen, & Peterson, 2004), which would constitute an adaptive plasticity in response to the expression of tics or habits, which, in turn, would help to inhibit them more easily. With the maturation of the frontal cortex during adolescence, this mechanism could gain strength, which explains the decrease in symptoms during adolescence and early adulthood. Among adults with persisting symptoms, this neuroplasticity could occur, but more research is needed.

These neurodevelopmental observations are compatible with CBT models (O'Connor, 2002). If the evolution and fluctuation of symptoms are related to a form of neuroplasticity, thus we propose that CBT will, in turn, improve symptoms as well as favoring neurophysiological changes corresponding to a normalization of cerebral function, a phenomenon that has recently been observed by our team (Branet, Hosatte-Ducassy, O'Connor, & Lavoie, 2010; Lavoie, Imbriglio, Stip, & O'Connor, 2011; Morand-Beaulieu et al., 2016; Morand-Beaulieu, Sauve, Blanchet, & Lavoie, 2015; O'Connor, 2005; O'Connor et al., 2001; O'Connor, Lavoie, Stip, Borgeat, & Laverdure, 2008).

Tics, Tourette's, and habits are not anyway caused exclusively by brain dysfunctions. There is no compelling evidence that people with Tourette's have neuropsychological alteration, except when it comes to organizing action and motor planning. Brain and behavior are a two-way traffic lane and it is conceivable that some brain anomaly is due to tic or habit suppression. Likewise, results from brain imaging and electrophysiology often fluctuate and it's likely that a subsample of people with persistent tics is susceptible to higher sensorimotor activation. In any case, our approach here is to put the emphasis on processes leading to tics, which can be considered common. An alternative model considers tics at least maintained by contingencies, where negative reinforcement could be an important cycle. This heightened vulnerability to sensorimotor activation may explain the lower threshold, but also heightened attention to sensory phenomena.

Cognitive and behavioral etiology

The presence of tics generates significant distress among certain individuals. These signs are distinguishable in terms of phobias, depression, social anxiety, self-image concerns, a decrease in self-esteem, relationship problems (Marcks, Berlin, Woods, & Davies, 2007; Woods & Marcks, 2005), the negative perception of peers, and social rejection (Anderson, Vu, Derby, Goris, & McLaughlin, 2002; Roane, Piazza, Cercone, & Grados, 2002). Also noticeable is a particular style of behavioral planning on a cognitive level. Thus, preliminary results from the STOP questionnaire (O'Connor, 2002) suggest that Tourette's syndrome would be defined by chronic overactivation, difficulty in staying focused, and the tendency to undertake many things at the same time (overactivity), as well as an increased investment in efforts related to motor function (overpreparation). These two components logically constitute the basic focus for therapy. In return, the treatment will sensibly lead to changes that impact on neuroplasticity.

Environmental and psychosocial etiology

Beyond the neurocognitive and behavioral origin of Tourette's syndrome, psychosocial observations are critical to embrace the full picture of symptom evolution. First, environmental factors such as the presence of an academic support and the quality of social interactions can influence symptom severity (Leclerc, Forget, & O'Connor, 2008). Moreover, behavioral approaches conceptualize tic or habit manifestations as being associated with principles of learning and the management of environmental contingencies (Azrin & Nunn, 1973). Within that perspective, tics are considered as an exaggerated response involving social operant conditioning. Consequently, the tic or habit manifestation would be more frequent when the individual receives attention, or when it allows him/her to avoid an unpleasant situation (Roane et al., 2002; Woods & Miltenberger, 2001). This theory can explain the simple fact that talking about vocal tics can cause an important increase in these manifestations. These hypotheses are partly based on observations that tics fluctuate in time, but they seem incomplete and today's research states that other factors may be involved.

In light of previous statements, a sound hypothesis of tic or habit onset requires linking the role of many interrelated causes. An interactive and multidimensional model appears to be more plausible than a model based on a unilateral and linear causality (APA, 2000; O'Connor, 2005; Woods & Miltenberger, 2001).

Social Impact and Consequences

Sensitivity to judgment

There have been several studies on the social consequences of ticking (Cavanna, David, Orth, & Robertson, 2012; Cavanna et al., 2013; Crossley & Eugenio Cavanna, 2013). Tic disorder clients tend to be sensitive to the judgment of others. The comorbidities present in tic disorder can interact with quality of life, and sometimes miscomprehension of tics and cognitive, behavioral, and social functions can interact with mood and relationship and influence quality of life and well-being. (Cavanna et al., 2012, 2013; Crossley & Eugenio Cavanna, 2013).

They are often over-concerned with self-image and fear the judgment of others, including, but not limited to, how their tic or habit looks to others (Thibert, Day, & Sandor, 1995), which leads them to feel dissatisfied with themselves. Tic disorder clients also scored higher than controls on items such as feeling ill at ease with others, and self-image dissatisfaction (O'Connor et al., 2001). Although there are no data to date on whether such sensitivity and self-focus could be the result of ticking, these concerns may easily feed into the ticking loop, and feed heightened physiological tension and dissatisfaction, as suggested by the fact that even persons with low awareness of their ticking and its visibility to others still display this heightened negative self-focus.

Current Treatment Options

Pharmacological treatments

Pharmacological treatments are one intervention of choice to help people with Tourette's syndrome. Various treatments have been proposed but the majority of prescription drugs, as much among adults as among children with Tourette's syndrome, show a variable response, even sometimes on the same individual. From the beginning, let us mention that no drug can lead to the complete remission of this syndrome, and the dosage is usually adjusted, according to the presence of the dominant tic or habit or behavioral symptoms. Because of the dominant hypothesis of tics as a problem of the motor circuits and the dopaminergic system, dopamine antagonist neuroleptics are routinely the main treatment. Therefore, many researchers have observed that pharmacological agents that trigger an increase (agonist) in dopaminergic functions will exacerbate tics (Golden, 1974; Riddle, Hardin, Towbin, Leckman, & Cohen, 1987), whereas those that bring a decrease (antagonist) of the dopaminergic action tend to reduce the tic or habit frequency (Lombroso et al., 1995; Shapiro et al., 1989).

According to the Canadian guidelines for the evidence-based treatment of tic disorders (Pringsheim et al., 2012), weak recommendations were made for children for the use of typical neuroleptics (pimozide, haloperidol, fluphenazine, metoclopramide) or atypical neuroleptics (risperidone, aripiprazole, olanzapine, quetiapine, ziprasidone, topiramate, baclofen), while other treatments such as botulinum toxin injections, tetrabenazine, and cannabinoids were weakly recommended for adults only. However, strong recommendations were made for the use of guanfacine and clonidine in children, which are both antihypertensive agents and alpha 2a agonists.

Typical antipsychotics may cause extra pyramidal signs, characterized by involuntary movements, impatience, a need to constantly move, and significant trembling among other symptoms. Atypical neuroleptic or drug combinations are reserved for more complex cases as well as in the presence of associated disorders. The effectiveness of atypical neuroleptics has progressively been proven to reduce tics, despite the possibility of significant long-term side effects, such as an increased risk of metabolic syndrome (i.e., hyperglycemia, weight gain, and diabetes). Other pharmacological agents (antidepressants or other neuroleptics) can provide positive results in reducing tics, but these results are often inconsistent and generally come from single cases and non-randomized trials (Pringsheim & Marras, 2009).

Managing tics and habits with the cognitive-behavioral approach

Azrin and Nunn (1973) were the first researchers to suggest that tics could be replaced by other behaviors. In their book *Habit Control in a Day* (1977) they suggested that the tic could be replaced by a response antagonistic to the tic tensing the opposite muscles and so impeding the tic. With practice the tic could be controlled until the tic was counter-conditioned and the urge even to tic disappeared. This same technique was applied to habits such as hair pulling, where the hands were kept occupied or in contact with a surface to impede movement to the hair or skin. The technique is termed habit reversal, and has been developed recently into a comprehensive behavioral intervention, CBIT, for tics where the main component is a competing response awareness and analysis of the stimulus and consequences of ticking in order to manage contingencies to reward non-ticking. There have been several studies affirming the validity of the CBIT approach and there are published manuals (Woods et al., 2012). Another approach particularly to managing habit disorders is the multi-modal comprehensive behavioral approach to controlling the habit, isolating and eliminating the stimulus signal for pulling whether it is sensory, cognitive, emotional, or perceptual (Falkenstein, Mouton-Odum, Mansueto, Goldfinger, & Haaga, 2015; Mansueto, Golomb, Thomas, & Stemberger, 1999). Currently, a CBT approach constitutes an effective line of treatment for adults with both tic disorders (McGuire, Piacentini et al., 2014; Wile & Pringsheim, 2013) and BFRB (Bloch et al., 2007; Gelinas & Gagnon, 2013; McGuire, Ung et al., 2014; Woods & Houghton, 2015). Another behavioral approach is exposure and response prevention, whereby the client tolerates the urge to tic whilst resisting the action of ticking (Verdellen, van de Griendt, Kriens, & van Oostrum, 2011). These approaches address the tic when it has occurred or when it is about to occur and do not look systematically at the processes leading up to and preceding the tic and tension onset as does the current CoPs approach. But the CoPs approach to management can be used in conjunction with the CBIT or comprehensive behavioral method or by itself. Another source of treatment is Keuthen and colleagues' (2012) inspiring use of dialectical behavior therapy and the addition of mindfulness to tic and habit management, and other authors have used the addition of ACT to supplement habit reversal therapy for habits (Christenson & Crow, 1996; Flessner, Busch, Heideman & Woods, 2008a; Flessner et al., 2008b, 2008c; Keuthen et al., 2007, 2012, 2015; Woods, Wetterneck, & Flessner, 2006).

The therapy proposed by our group is based on the CoPs model, which aims at regulating the high level of sensorimotor activation present in these populations and preventing the buildup of tension that leads to tic bursts or to the habit disorder (Lavoie, Leclerc, & O'Connor, 2013; O'Connor, 2002; O'Connor, Lavoie, Blanchet, & St-Pierre-Delorme, 2015). Although empirical studies are limited, the

CoPs approach also has shown efficacy. Its effectiveness in treating adults affected by either disorder has been replicated (O'Connor et al., 2001, 2009, 2015). Over the past 10 years, our group has conducted a number of studies exploring the cognitive-behavioral and psychophysiological manifestations of motor activation in Tourette's syndrome/tic disorder with the aim of linking the multi-level processes evoking tic onset with behavioral management procedures (Lavoie et al., 2013; Leclerc et al., 2008; O'Connor, 2005; O'Connor et al., 2005, 2008, 2009; Thibault, 2009). These experimental and clinical findings have led to elaboration of a cognitive-behavioral/psychophysiological model of treatment (Lavoie et al., 2013; O'Connor et al., 2015), which proposes: (a) an overactive style of planning that prevents optimal preparation for action; (b) this style leads to problems regulating arousal/inhibition processes particularly under circumstances where regulation is open-looped, controlled, and has unpredictable parameters; (c) such high levels of motor activation create tension and frustration and are likely to evoke ticking; (d) hence a CBT package, which addresses the cognitive psychophysiological sources of motor activation reducing background tension and preventing tic onset. Rather than target solely the tic implicated muscle in a competing response antagonistic to the tic, an important additional component in our CBT program is a modification of excessive overall motor activation, by targeting cognitive and behavioral/physiological sources creating tension. There were also significant changes post-treatment in measures of self-esteem, anxiety, depression, and style of planning action (O'Connor et al., 2001). More recent clinical trials have found CoPs effective for habit disorder (O'Connor et al., 2017.).

Therapist checklist for information on tics and habits

The client understands what constitutes a tic or a habit	Yes / No ❏ ❏
The client understands recent findings on the nature of tics and habits	Yes / No ❏ ❏
The client understands how tension maintains tics and habits and at the same time how tics and habits give relief from tension	Yes / No ❏ ❏
The client understands the model of the program addressing downstream processes, the structure, and the evolution of the program	Yes / No ❏ ❏
The client understands that the program progresses in stages each addressing different psychophysiological processes leading up to the tic or habit	Yes / No ❏ ❏
The client understands the model and how we address flexibility in tension, preparation, and thought	Yes / No ❏ ❏
The client chose a good metaphor to mark to progress	Yes / No ❏ ❏
The client understands that the program is cumulative and progresses stage by stage	Yes / No ❏ ❏

2

Evaluation and Assessment

In this chapter we define tics and habits, describe criteria and provide guidelines for identifying problematic tics and habits,. We explain the use of scales to measure the distress and severity associated with tics and habits, and tabulate illustrations on how to sort out the difference between tics and habits. We discuss other scales measuring style of action and assessing degree of beliefs about tics or habits, which could influence progress.

Evaluation and Assessment: What are Tics and Habits?

Simple tics are defined as repetitive non-voluntary contractions of functionally related groups of skeletal muscles in one or more parts of the body including blinking, cheek twitches, head or knee jerks, and shoulder shrugs. Complex tics involve several movements or muscles often comprising a sequence of several different muscle contractions. There has been controversy about current criteria for Tourette's syndrome, but the diagnosis is currently dichotomous, not dimensional, and depends crucially on the existence of a phonic tic. However, clinician consensus suggests a continuum of severity, in particular between chronic motor tic disorder and Tourette's disorder. This division is really historical dating from the initial observation, at the time, of only severe cases with phonic tics, but tic disorder can be just as severe as Tourette's disorder.

Here we consider tic disorder and Tourette's disorder on a continuum with habit disorder and they are all equally responsive to the program.

Body focused repetitive behaviors (BFRBs) are tic-related disorders, which we term here habit disorders, which encompass symptoms that are directed toward the body, in reaction to feelings of discomfort. Habit disorders may take the form of self-inflicted repetitive actions such as nail biting, hair pulling, head slapping, face scratching, teeth grinding, and tense–release hand gripping cycles. There is a clear benefit in distinguishing between tic disorder and habit disorders, for the reason that the relationship between these two entities is sometimes clinically unclear and because the presence of complex movements in habit disorder can often be confused with complex tics. A scientific method of differentiating these two groups is to compare directly their event-related brain activity by contrasting

Managing Tic and Habit Disorders: A Cognitive Psychophysiological Approach with Acceptance Strategies, First Edition. Kieron P O'Connor, Marc E Lavoie, and Benjamin Schoendorff.
© 2017 John Wiley & Sons, Ltd. Published 2017 by John Wiley & Sons, Ltd.
Companion Website: www.wiley.com/go/oconnor/managingticandhabitdsorders

tasks with different levels of motor demand. For instance, O'Connor et al. (2005) reported that people with tic disorder and habit disorder patients both failed to adequately adjust their hand responses to automated or controlled movements. More precisely, people with tic disorders had the most severe impairment in synchronizing their cerebral activity with their actual hand response time, followed by the people with habit disorder and the non-clinical control groups. These findings give support to a dimensional model of classification, with habit disorder falling between tic disorder and non-clinical controls along a continuum of motor arousal. Key distinguishing factors between tics and habits are: degree of awareness, goal of action, motivation, and emotional triggers. There is a range of habit subtypes, the most frequent being: hair pulling, chewing, skin picking, and nail biting. There may be idiosyncratic varieties of behavior that still form part of the spectrum, such as symmetry movements or joint cracking, and the client may have yet another non-specified variety of behavior that will nonetheless meet the criteria (see Table 2.1).

It is important the client and therapist compile a complete list of tics and habits both current and past. This can be achieved by therapist and client filling in the interview schedule shown in Tables 2.2 and 2.3. We also need to decide on what is initially a clinically significant problem or a tic problem. Sometimes people link tics and habits with obsessive-compulsive disorder (OCD) since these disorders seem similar—both seeming to involve ritualized actions. But they are different. OCD involves engaging in compulsive actions or mental rituals in response to intrusive thoughts so as to alleviate the anxiety that these thoughts generate. Some people may have both tics and OCD but they are distinct disorders. Although the program addresses both tics and habits, which we consider part of the same spectrum, we do not consider obsessions, which require a different approach to management from tics and habits (see O'Connor and Aardema, 2012), although we do provide guidelines (Tables 2.4–2.6) to help distinguish obsessions from habits.

Evaluating the Severity of Tics and Habits and Their Impact on the Client's Life

Tourette's disorder symptom severity can be assessed with the Tourette Syndrome Global Scale (TSGS; Harcherik, Leckman, Detlor, & Cohen, 1984). The first TSGS factor rates the nature of the tic (i.e., motor or phonic), while the second scale rates the tic complexity. A third scale assesses functional impairment, including behavioral, learning, motor restlessness, and occupational problems. The inter-rater reliability of the TSGS global score was found to be very good ($k = 0.77$, $P < 0.001$).

Currently, the gold standard is based on the use of the Yale Global Tic Severity Scale (YGTSS; Leckman et al., 1989) to establish a comprehensive picture of the tics. The YGTSS is derived in part from the TSGS, and is a scale completed by the clinician to quantify the severity of the symptoms, including their frequency, their duration, their intensity, and their complexity. The subscales assess

Table 2.1 Classification of tics according to the International Statistical Classification of Diseases and Related Health Problems Version 10 (ICD-X) and the Diagnostic and Statistical Manual of Mental Disorders Version 5 (DSM-5)

	ICD-X	DSM-V
Provisional tic disorder	Tic corresponds to general criterion, but persists no longer than 12 months (F95.0)	Presence of one or more motor tics or vocal tics for less than 12 months in a row and the tic must have started before the age of 18 (307.21)
Persistent (chronic) motor or vocal tic disorder	Characterized by the presence of exclusively motor or vocal tics persisting more than 1 year (F95.1)	Presence of one or more motor tics or vocal tics, but not both for less than 12 months in a row and the tic must have started before the age of 18 (307.22)
Gilles de la Tourette	Characterized by multiple motor tics and at least one vocal tic (F95.2)	Presence of two or more motor tics and at least one vocal tic for at least 1 year and must have started before the age of 18 (307.23)
Unspecified tic disorder	Residual category where tic is undefined (F95.9)	Presence of symptoms characteristic of a tic disorder that does not meet the full criteria for a tic disorder (307.20)
Trichotillomania	A disorder characterized by repetitive pulling out of one's hair resulting in noticeable hair loss; the individual experiences a rising subjective sense of tension before pulling out the hair and a sense of gratification or relief when pulling out the hair (F63.3)	Recurrent pulling out of one's hair, resulting in hair loss. Repeated attempts to decrease or stop hair pulling. The hair pulling causes clinically significant distress or impairment in social, occupational, or other important areas of functioning (312.39)
Excoriation disorder	Not present in the ICD-X	Excoriation (skin picking) disorder is characterized by recurrent skin picking resulting in skin lesions. Individuals with excoriation disorder must have made repeated attempts to decrease or stop the skin picking, which must cause clinically significant distress or impairment in social, occupational, or other important areas of functioning (698.4)

separately the tics and vocal tics, and can also generate combined scores. The YGTSS has a good internal consistency, inter-rater reliability, and an acceptable validity. Convergent validity of the motor and phonic tic factors showed strong correlations with the corresponding TSGS, with correlations ranging from $r = 0.86$ to $r = 0.91$ (Leckman et al., 1989).

To assess habit disorder, we propose an adaptation of the TSGS to assess the presence of habit disorders. In these adapted versions of both questionnaires, the

Table 2.2 Therapist interview schedule for assessing tic and habit severity

B] Description of the problem—*tic*

- *Do you have certain involuntary movements of one or more muscles groups, have a repetitive sensation that may arise, the urge to say words, phrases, swearing, to clear your throat, make certain noises, or to breathe in a certain repetitive manner or have something stuck in your head, like a song, a word, or a phrase that you can't get rid of? Typically this type of movement, sensation, or noise is associated with an increase in tension and it is produced against your will. This is not like a habit that you can control. Even if you are able to suppress it for a certain period of time, you may feel you will have to let it out sometimes. This type of movement is also not like habits that you are conscious of like pulling out hairs or biting your nails, even if the habit is automatic.*

Tics (identify if it is a motor, mental, sensory, or vocal tic and its location on the body)	Type of tic (simple, complex,. . .)	Frequency (number of times/hr)

1) (If there are many tics at the same time):
   - *Which one is the most visible?* _____
   - *Which one is the most disturbing?* _____
   - *If you had a choice, which one would you like to resolve the most?* _____
2) *Age of onset of the first tic symptoms experienced :*_____
3) *Is the occurrence of the tic(s) linked to a particular event?* (accident, intoxication)
   ❑ yes → which one?:_____
   _____
   ❑ no
4) *Is there a physical/neurological reason that can explain your tic(s)?*
   ❑ yes → which one?:_____
   _____
   ❑ no
5) *Have you ever had a neurological exam?*
   ❑ Yes
   ❑ no
6) *Have you ever received treatment for your tic(s)?*_____
   _____
7) *Has the tic(s) changed over time (e.g., in severity, in occurrence)?*
   ❑ yes → define:_____
   _____
   _____
   ❑ no

(continued)

8) *When does the tic(s) occur?*
   ❑ always
   ❑ under stress (or fatigue/tiredness)
   ❑ other situations: _____

9) *Presence of a sensation before the tics occur (e.g., a feeling, urge, itch)?*
   ❑ yes → define: _____
   _____
   ❑ no

10) *Presence of an emotion before the tic(s) occur (e.g., anxiety, frustration)?*
   ❑ yes → define: _____
   _____
   ❑ no

11) *Visibility of the tic(s):*
   *Tic:*_____
   ❑ not visible at all
   ❑ a little visible
   ❑ very visible
   *Tic:*_____
   ❑ not visible at all
   ❑ a little visible
   ❑ very visible
   *Tic:*_____
   ❑ not visible at all
   ❑ a little visible
   ❑ very visible
   *Tic:*_____
   ❑ not visible at all
   ❑ a little visible
   ❑ very visible

12) *Ability to suppress/control the tic(s):*
   ❑ always
   ❑ often
   ❑ sometimes
   If yes → how? _____
   → duration (min.)?_____
   ❑ never

13) *Do you sometimes hide your tic(s)?* (e.g., with another movement or with clothes)
   ❑ yes → define:_____
   _____
   ❑ no

14) *Impact of the tic(s) on:*
   Work:
   ❑ none
   ❑ a little
   ❑ a lot
   Interpersonal relationships:
   ❑ none
   ❑ a little
   ❑ a lot
   Activities:
   ❑ none
   ❑ a little
   ❑ a lot
   Other:_____
   ❑ none
   ❑ a little
   ❑ a lot

(continued)

Table 2.2 (Continued)

C] Description of habit disorder

1) *Do you have or have you ever had a habit disorder (involuntary destructive habit to calm a tension) like, for example, to pull out your hair, to grind your teeth, to scratch your skin, or to bite your nails?*
　❑ no → question # 5
　❑ yes → define:

Habit disorder(s) (identify which one)	Frequency (number of times/day)

2) *Since when have you had this habit (age)?* _____

3) *Degree of severity?* _____
_____

4) *Treatment?* _____
_____

5) *Do you have or have you ever had impulsive behaviors like gambling, starting fires in a compulsive manner, stealing in a compulsive manner, or indiscreet sexual behaviors?*
　❑ no → question # 9
　❑ yes → define: _____
_____

6) *Since when have you had these impulsive behaviors? (age)?* _____

7) *Degree of severity?* _____
_____

8) *Treatment?* _____
_____

9) *Do you have or have you ever had any other problems like, for example, hyperactivity or an attention disorder?* (as a child, adolescent or adult)
　❑ no → question # 13
　❑ yes → define: _____
_____

10) *Since when (age)?* _____

11) *Degree of severity?* _____
_____

(continued)

12) *Treatment?*_____
_____

13) *Which of these problems is the most disturbing?*
  ❑ tic
  ❑ habit disorder
  ❑ impulsive behavior
  ❑ hyperactivity, attention disorder
  ❑ others → define:_____

14) *Other family members with similar problems (tic or habit disorder)?*
  ❑ husband/wife
→ define:_____
_____
→ treatment:_____
  ❑ children
→ define:_____
_____
→ treatment:_____
  ❑ father/mother
→ define:_____
_____
→ treatment:_____
  ❑ brother/sister
→ define:_____
_____
→ treatment:_____
  ❑ grandfather/grandmother
define:_____
_____
→ treatment:_____
  ❑ uncle/aunt
define:_____
_____
→ treatment:_____
  ❑ cousin → define:_____
_____
→ treatment:_____

D] Description of the problem—*other difficulties*

1) *Beside the symptoms we've just talked about, do you have any other psychological or emotional difficulties for which you would like to seek help?*
  ❑ no → question # 3.
  ❑ yes→ which one? _____

2) *What bothers you the most between the tics or the habit disorder and this other difficulty?*
  ❑ tics
  ❑ habit disorder
  ❑ other difficulty
  ● For a total of 100%, what percentage do you attribute to the compulsions/obsessions and to this other difficulty?
    a. tics: _____%
    b. habit disorder: _____%
    c. other difficulty: _____%
  ❑ *Presently do you have a physical health problem?*
  ❑ no
  ❑ yes
→ To what extent could this problem prevent you from participating in the program? _____
_____
_____

  ❑ → Do you think this problem is associated with your tics?

Table 2.3 Evaluation of actual life functioning for tics and habits (adapted from DSM-IV-TR)

Code: .... **Date:** .... **Evaluator:** ....

Evaluate the actual life functioning of the patient (last 14 days) in each domain of his life on the following scale. For example, *Could you describe to me how your tic or habit symptoms have influenced your life in the last two weeks?* Question, if necessary, to identify other elements. Score the highest interference mentioned. e.g., "It prevents me from moving forward and I often forget important things. I have been reprimanded because of that" → 5.

1 No problem in this domain.

3 The patient functions well in this domain but the tics or habits prevent him or her from moving forward or taking advantage of the situation (e.g., doesn't take advantage of occasion to advance, lack of initiative, complains about the tics, which spoil positive events, less available for spouse or children).

5 The functioning of the client is undermined in this domain, most of the time, but he or she is still functional (e.g., difficulty in studying, difficulty at work (relationships, attention, etc.), intermittent family/spouse conflicts because of the tics or of associated mood).

7 The client still functions in this domain but with some difficulties or important lack (e.g., reduced academic productivity, reduced performance at work, important deterioration of family relationships, no sexual activity).

9 The client experiments severe difficulties in functioning in this domain, does not function, or functions only a little (e.g., quit studying, sick, quit or lost job, spousal relationship in peril).

A) Job, professional activity, study, or usual occupation

_____

1	2	3	4	5	6	7	8	9	10
No problem									Severe difficulties

B) Spousal or romantic relationships and family life

_____

1	2	3	4	5	6	7	8	9	10
No problem									Severe difficulties

C) Hobby, spare time, holidays, and daily activities (cleaning, running errands, etc.)

_____

1	2	3	4	5	6	7	8	9	10
No problem									Severe difficulties

Table 2.4 Differential diagnosis

Tics	Stereotypes	Habit disorder	Obsessions/compulsions
Form			
• Selected muscle group • Saccadic • Location can change	• Whole trunk or body • Rhythmic • Fixed form and location	• Involve auto-mutilation • Sequenced flow • Stable sequence	• Complex behaviors • Follow action plan • Repetitive behavior
Awareness			
• Minimal or zero	• Some	• Medium	• Full
Emotion			
• Frustration, impatience, boredom	• Preoccupation	• Complex moods (guilt, depression)	• Anxiety
Triggers			
• Situation or activities • Tension	• Internal state • Movement feedback	• Mood and situation • Need for stimulation	• Obsessional fear • Harm reduction
Treatment			
• Relaxation, habit reversal	• Operant counter-conditioning	• Cognitive and behavior therapy	• Exposure and response prevention

Table 2.5 Example of similar complex mental tics and obsessional compulsions

Complex mental tics	Obsessional compulsions
• Looking or enveloping an object • Repeating phrases • Mental games • Playful thoughts • Running through mental scenes for fun • Copying what others would do or say • Saying or doing because it's stimulating or because it can't be inhibited • Counting words on a sign	• Intentional staring to check • Verbal repetition of a ritual • Aversive flashes or images • Disturbing ideas • Repeating events mentally to check for errors • Stereotyped response due to OCD rules • Saying or doing to ward off bad luck • Counting for superstitious reasons

word "tic" was replaced by the word "habit." These questionnaires were adapted to quantify both tics and habits on the same metric uniformly. This adaptation has been validated in prior research by our group (O'Connor et al., 2017).

We prefer the TSGS since it is multidimensional, measuring tics and behavioral activation, and also it is sensitive to change. The full versions of these assessment instruments and other shorter tic scales are given in the references. Here, we enclose our own shorter assessment form to assess severity of the tics and habits and to measure frequency intensity and distress adapted from our studies, adapted to our program. This instrument measures: history, habit characteristics,

Table 2.6 Questionnaire for distinguishing obsessive-compulsive disorder from obsessive-compulsive disorder with Tourette's syndrome (inspired by George et al., 1993).

	Yes	No	Tourette's or OCD
1. Do you have urges to touch things?	❏	❏	Tourette's
2. Do you sometimes suddenly feel the urge to touch yourself or your bodily parts?	❏	❏	Tourette's
3. Do you have impulses to hurt yourself?	❏	❏	Tourette's
4. If you answered yes to the above question, is it because of feelings of guilt or uncleanliness?	❏	❏	OCD
5. Do you sometime have to repeat things several times, for no reason?	❏	❏	OCD
6. Do you sometime have a profound urge to explore things in your environment?	❏	❏	Tourette's
7. If you have sudden urges of any kind, are they preceded by thoughts of guilt or uncleanliness?	❏	❏	OCD
8. When you act on your urges, do you feel guilty?	❏	❏	OCD
9. Do you sometime have the urge to harm yourself or others?	❏	❏	OCD
10. Do your compulsions or urges arise from nowhere?	❏	❏	OCD
11. Do you feel a need to imitate other people?	❏	❏	Tourette's
12. Do dirty words or thoughts come into your head when you are thinking about other things?	❏	❏	OCD
13. Do bloody or violent scenes pop into your head when you are thinking about other things?	❏	❏	Tourette's
14. Do you feel a need to do other things that you know will cause you bodily harm, such as touching hot objects or hitting yourself?	❏	❏	Tourette's
15. Have you worried about blurting out an obscenity or a phrase or doing something sexual (like exposing yourself) in public?	❏	❏	Tourette's

type of tic, and everyday dysfunction on a scale adapted from the DSM-IV (Table 2.3), but we recommend a full diagnostic interview. It would be useful to measure comorbidities using a structured interview to help in deciding priorities. We also include tables to distinguish between tics and habits (see Table 2.7), and to distinguish tics from non-tic twitches and habits from trivial twiddles, to ensure the problem is clinically significant (see Tables 2.8 and Table 2.9).

We also propose the Massachusetts General Hospital Hair Pulling Scale (MGH-HPS; Keuthen et al., 1995) and skin picking scale to assess habit disorder severity (Keuthen et al., 2001). The MGH-HPS is a 7-point scale measuring severity of hair pulling symptoms, which has been adapted to nail biting, skin scratching, and skin picking. We provide below an adapted checklist for assessing: hair pulling, nail biting, skin picking, skin scratching, and other non-specified habit disorders.

Table 2.7 Distinguishing tic disorders and habit disorders

Tic disorder	Habit disorder
Complex movement or simple movement, but involving muscles in a sequence	Complex movement involving several body parts
All parts of the body can be involved	Movement generally involves hand functions
Generally goal is internal to alleviate sensation	Goal in carrying out habit is to alleviate mood
Emotions are generally anxiety and frustration	Linked to emotion and difficulty regulating emotions
Generally no emotions post-treatment, except relief from tension	Positive and negative emotions present pre- and post-habit
No intent to self-mutilate	Involve self-mutilation/destruction of hair, skin, nails, etc.
Degree of awareness varies and it is incomplete	Can be performed consciously or automatically
Automatic reflexlike	Elements uncontrollable but involved controlled muscles
Decrease tension	Decrease emotion

Table 2.8 Different criteria for identifying between habit disorders and harmless habits such as twiddles

Habit disorder	Twiddles
Self-destructive acts with negative impact on body parts	Minor motor movements, usually involving hands, legs, arms, and complex voluntary sequences, which can be controlled by awareness or countermanding, for example:
The person feels obliged to perform and cannot easily control; the habit functions in controlling mood	• Playing with paper clip • Passing hand through hair
Related to mood regulation	• Grooming behavior • Smooching or smacking lips
Causes severe distress and impairment	• Turning up nose • Rotating thumbs • Pushing thumbs over nails

Note: Twitches and twiddles can of course become tics and habits if they develop and so change criteria from the right hand to the left hand column.

We provide tables listing clinical differences between BFRBs and tics and OCD compulsions (Tables 2.7–2.9). Prior studies found correlations between TSGS scores rating habits and the MGH-HPS ($r = 0.49$, $P < 0.05$), as well as the MGH scales adapted for nail biting and skin picking ($r = 0.52$, $P < 0.05$) (O'Connor et al., 2017). Another measure, not included here, but referred to, is the Milwaukee hair pulling scale, which differentiates automatic and controlled pulling (Flessner

Table 2.9 Differentiating tic or habit disorders from harmless habits such as twitches, which can be easily controlled

Tic or habit	Twitches
Repetitive involuntary or semi-voluntary of one or several muscles causing distress/dysfunction	Occasional involuntary spasm not repetitive, benign transient, and non-aversive
Involves a sequences or series	A spasm due to unusual stretching
Always associated with high tension	Blinking in strong sunlight
Releases tension as part of reinforcement cycle	Flinching when hearing loud sound
Chronic and repetitive	Shivering with cold
	Muscle twitching when fatigued
	Abrupt jerking when stretching
	Occasional jerks after movement

et al., 2008c). However, this distinction is controversial since it seems all habit disorders contain some elements of conscious and unconscious actions.

Assessing Style of Planning and Thinking and Beliefs about Tics or Habits

As part of our research program, we also developed a style of planning question-naire (STOP) that measures style of planning in everyday life. The STOP has now been validated and has good reliability and discriminates between tic disorder and controls (O'Connor, 2005; O'Connor et al., 2015). Its three main factors are: overactivity, overpreparation, and overcomplication in planning action. The results suggest that all tic and habit disorders show elevated scores compared with others in particular on the first two factors. In addition, the overactivity subscale correlates highly with the TSGS global subscale of motor restlessness. This STOP measure becomes very important in achieving the cognitive and behavioral flexibility of style of action explored in detail in Chapter 5. Other scales including the short form of the tics scale and the premonitory urges in Tourette's scale (PUTS) are given in the references.

   An important part of the assessment process is evaluating the way the client judges and thinks about his or her tic. It is important also to measure the longstanding beliefs the client has about his or her tic that may be lurking in the background, and we include a form on thinking about tics, which we have validated as a measure of how thoughts can influence the tic, and which we address in our program. The Thinking about Tics questionnaire (THAT) has been validated as a valid and reliable measure of anticipations in tic and habit disorders. It measures three factors: whether the client's tics will interfere with his or her activities; the extent to which the client anticipates the arrival

Table 2.10 Version 1—Hair pulling scale (adapted from Keuthen et al., 2007; Harcherik et al., 1984)

Name: _____   Date: _____

Instructions: Answer each question, according to your behaviours and/or feelings when you typically pull your hair.

You typically may or may not have the urge to pull your hair even if you do not act on it.

For the next three questions, rate only the urges to pull your hair

1) *Frequency of urges.* On an average day, how often did you feel the urge to pull your hair? Number of times: _____

2) *Intensity of urges.* On an average day, how intense or "strong" were the urges to pull your hair? Very strong; strong; modest; weak _____

_____

3) *Ability to control urges.* On an average day, how much control do you have over the urges to pull your hair? Strong control; some control; no control _____

For the next three questions, rate only the actual hair pulling

4) *Frequency of hair pulling.* On an average day, how often did you actually pull your hair? Number of times:_____

5) *Complexity of hair pulling.* On an average day what actions are involved in your hair pulling? Describe sequence of moves

_____

_____

6) *Control over hair pulling.* On an average day, how often were you successful at actually stopping yourself from pulling your hair? Very successful; somewhat successful,unsuccess ful_____

7) *Tensions during pulling.* On an average day, in which parts of your body do you detect tension? Tension in_____

_____

8) *Moods associated with hair pulling.* Hair pulling can involve several emotions at the before, during, and after hair pulling. During the past week, how did your hair pulling make you feel: before hair pulling?_____during hair pulling? _____after hair pulling_?

of the tic; and the extent to which the client gives themselves permission to tic. The anticipation scale and the interference scale do change post-treatment, indicating that these scales are affected by treatment (O'Connor et al., 2014). The THAT can be discussed with the client and permits an initial focus on the ways that thinking about the tic or habit influence onset. The aim of the STOP and the THAT is to stimulate at the onset awareness in the clients that the way they think about their own tics and the way they plan their actions are relevant to the tic, as they will feature strongly in our program (Tables 2.15 and 2.16).

Table 2.11 Version 2—Nail biting scale (adapted from Keuthen et al., 2007; Harcherik et al., 1984)

Name: _____   Date: _____

Instructions: Answer each question, according to your behaviours and/or feelings when you typically bite your nails.

You typically may or may not have the urge to bite your nails even if you do not act on it.

For the next three questions, rate only the urges to bite your nails

1) *Frequency of urges.* On an average day, how often did you feel the urge to bite your nails? Number of times _____

2) *Intensity of urges.* On an average day, how intense or "strong" were the urges to bite your nails? Very strong; strong; modest; weak _____

_____

3) *Ability to control urges.* On an average day, how much control do you have over the urges to bite your nails? Strong control; some control; no control_____
_____

For the next three questions, rate only the actual nail biting

4) *Frequency of nail biting.* On an average day, how often did you actually bite your nails? Number of times_____

5) Complexity of nail biting. On an average day what actions are involved in your hair pulling? Describe sequence of moves _____
_____

6) *Control over nail biting.* On an average day, how often were you successful at actually stopping yourself from biting your nails? Very successful; somewhat successful, unsuccessful

_____

7) *Tensions during nail biting.* On an average day, in which parts of your body do you detect tension? Tension in :_____

8) *Moods associated with nail biting.* Nail biting can involve several emotions at the before, during, and after biting. During the past week, how did your nail biting make you feel: Before nail biting?_____during nail biting?_____after nail biting?_____

The goal of completing these evaluations is to record tics or habits, degree of distress, and an element surrounding the tic or habit to decide on:

1) Whether the client has a clinically significant problem.
2) The type of tic or habit and its severity and its impact on life.
3) Whether there are other problems or obstacles to pursuing the program.
4) Whether the client's history suggests further screening for medical problem.
5) Style of action—helps determine whether the client has a tic or habit profile.
6) Thinking about tics underlies the importance of thinking.
7) The evaluation also gives therapist and client insight into the nature and priority of their problem in preparation for the program.

Table 2.12 Version 3—Scratching scale (adapted from Harcherik 1984; Keuthen et al., 2007)

Name: _____   Date: _____

Instructions: Answer each question, according to your behaviours and/or feelings when you typically scratch.
You typically may or may not have the urge to scratch even if you do not act on it.

For the next three questions, rate only the urges to scratch

1) *Frequency of urges.* On an average day, how often did you feel the urge to scratch? Number of times

2) *Intensity of urges.* On an average day, how intense or "strong" were the urges to scratch? Very strong; moderately strong; weak; no urge

3) *Ability to control urges.* On an average day, how much control do you have over the urges to scratch? Strong control; somewhat control; weak control; no control:

_____
_____
_____

For the next three questions, rate only the actual scratching

4) *Frequency of scratching.* On an average day, how often did you actually scratch? Number of times_____

5) *Complexity of scratching.* On an average day what is the sequence of actions involved in scratching? Describe the sequence of moves: _____
_____
_____

6) *Control over scratching.* On an average day, how often were you successful at actually stopping yourself from scratching? Very successful; somewhat successful, unsuccessful

_____

7) *Tensions during scratching.* On an average day, in which parts of your body do you detect tension? Tension in:

_____

Moods associated with scratching

8) *Moods associated with scratching.* Scratching can involve several emotions at the before, during, and after scratching. During the past week, how did you feel: before scratching?_____during scratching?_____after scratching? _____
_____
_____

Table 2.13 Version 4—Skin picking scale (adapted from Keuthen et al., 2007; Harcherik et al 1984)

Name: _____   Date: _____

Instructions: Answer each question, according to your behaviours and/or feelings when you typically skin pick.
You typically may or may not have the urge to skin pick even if you do not act on it.

For the next three questions, rate only the urges to skin pick

1) *Frequency of urges.* On an average day, how often did you feel the urge to skin pick? Number of times

2) *Intensity of urges.* On an average day, how intense or "strong" were the urges to skin pick? Very strong; moderately strong; weak; no urge

3) *Ability to control urges.* On an average day, how much control do you have over the urges to skin pick? Strong control; somewhat control; weak control; no control :_____

For the next three questions, rate only the actual skin picking

4) *Frequency of skin picking.* On an average day, how often did you actually skin pick? Number of times_____

5) *Complexity of skin picking.* On an average day what is the sequence of actions involved in skin picking? Describe the sequence of moves: _____

Control over skin picking. On an average day, how often were you successful at actually stopping yourself from skin picking? Very successful; somewhat successful, unsuccessful

---

6) *Tensions during skin picking.* On an average day, in which parts of your body do you detect tension? Tension in:

Moods associated with skin picking

7) *Moods associated with skin picking.* Skin picking can involve several emotions at the before, during, and after skin picking. During the past week, how did you feel: before skin picking?_____during skin picking?_____after skin picking?

Table 2.14 Version 5—Individual personalized habits scale (adapted from Harcherik et al., 1984; Keuthen et al., 2007)

Name: _____   Date: _____

Instructions: Answer each question, according to your behaviours and/or feelings when you typically _____ (fill in personalized habit disorder)

If you typically may or may not have the urge to _____ even if you do not act on it

_____
_____

For the next three questions, rate only the urges to _____

Frequency of urges. On an average day, how often did you feel the urge to _____?
Number of times_____

Intensity of urges. On an average day, how intense or "strong" were the urges to_____?
Very strong; moderately strong; weak; none_____

Ability to control urges. On an average day, how much control do you have over the urges
to_____? Very strong control; somewhat control; weak control, no
control_____

For the next three questions, rate only the actual _____

Frequency of_____. On an average day, how often did you actually_____? Number
of times_____

Complexity of_____. On an average day what actions are involved in your _____?
Describe sequence of moves _____
_____

Control over _____. On an average day, how often were you successful at actually
stopping yourself from _____? Very successful; somewhat successful, unsuccessful
_____

Tensions during _____. On an average day, in which parts of your body do you detect
tension? Tension in_____

---

*Moods associated with _____. _____*can involve several emotions at the before
during and after. During the past week, how did your _____make you feel?__
before_____during_____after_____
_____

Table 2.15 Style of planning (STOP) (from O'Connor et al., 2015)

Below are listed examples of activities you are likely to encounter during the day. We ask you to indicate how you would anticipate dealing with these situations by marking a vertical line at right angles to the horizontal line in between the two extreme approaches to the problem.

If your approach most clearly resembles the right option, place a vertical line as far as possible to the right; if it clearly resembles the left, place your line to the far left. If your preference is towards one option, but lies somewhere in between the two alternatives, place your line at the appropriate point along the right or left section of the horizontal line.

If you would be equally likely to use both approaches with no preference, then place the line midway.

Here is an example:

| 1. You are shopping in a supermarket and a person in front of you is slow and holding up the queue. Is your immediate reaction to feel: |
| .... \| .... |
| Very impatient   Very sympathetic |

1) You are shopping in a supermarket and a person in front of you is slow and holding up the queue. Is your immediate reaction to feel:

.... | ....   OA

Very impatient   Very sympathetic

2) Do you find you overprepare for a task and put in more effort than is really required?

.... | ....   OP

All the time   Never

3) When you carry out an assignment, do you:

.... | ....   OP

Prepare well in advance   Wait until the last minute to prepare

4) You are required to sit still for 15 minutes. Is this:

.... | ....   OA

Impossible   No problem

5) When planning your agenda for a day, do you:

.... | ....   OA

Have a realistic idea of how much you can achieve   Cram as much activity
                                                                           in as you can

6) You anticipate that some unfamiliar or unknown event is likely to occur. Do you:

.... | ....   OP

Tense up immediately   Take it in your stride

7) When doing an activity, are you more frequently:

.... | ....   OA

Impatient to get ahead and finish   Enjoying just doing the job

8) Do you have the impression that you're overpreparing for a task and deploying more effort than necessary?

.... | ....   OP

Always   Never

9) When estimating the length of time a job takes, do you more often:

.... | ....   OA

Overestimate how much you can do   Underestimate how much
                                                                        you can do

(continued)

10) Do you have a tendency to overcomplicate what to others seem straightforward plans?

. . . . | . . . . ☐ OC

Always   Never

11) When planning a job, do you imagine all sorts of unforeseen eventualities that might happen and make the job seem more difficult?

. . . . | . . . . ☐ OC

Always   Never

12) When planning a job, are you more likely to:

. . . . | . . . . ☐ OC

Elaborate each stage in detail beforehand   Stick with a general idea of
                                                      what is required

13) Do you find yourself getting sidetracked in the middle of your tasks, which makes you go to unnecessary effort

. . . . | . . . . ☐ OC

Always   Never

14) When you're concentrating on a task, are you:

. . . . | . . . . ☐ OC

Frequently distracted   Easily capable of maintaining your attention

15) When you carry out an assignment, do you:

. . . . | . . . . ☐ OP

Prepare yourself early   Wait until the last second

OA stands for overactive, OP stands for overprepared, and OC stands for overcomplication.

Table 2.16 Thinking about Tics Inventory form (THAT)

Table X 12-item loading on the three scales of the Thinking About Tics Inventory				
Item number	Item	Interference 1	Anticipation 2	Permission 3
1	Anticipating that you might tic	❑	❑	❑
2	Thinking in general about your tics	❑	❑	❑
4	The idea that you must tic to feel relief	❑	❑	❑
5	Talking about your tics	❑	❑	❑
6	Knowing that you will be with people who expect you to have tics	❑	❑	❑
7	Wondering if your tics will interfere with your activities	❑	❑	❑
10	Knowing that you have the permission to tic	❑	❑	❑
15	Thinking that the tics spoil your image	❑	❑	❑
16	Thinking that you appear odd and different due to your tics	❑	❑	❑
20	Observing someone else tic	❑	❑	❑
21	Thinking that your tics make you look bad	❑	❑	❑
22	Noticing that you have not ticked in a while	❑	❑	❑

Items 1, 2, 3, 4, 5, 22 (anticipation); items 7, 15, 16, 21 (interference); items 3, 6, 10, 20 (permission).

Therapist checklist for evaluation

Client and therapist completed the assessment forms	Yes / No ❏ ❏
Client listed all tics and habits as well as severity and distress depending on tic or habit (completed relevant versions of habit disorder scales)	Yes / No ❏ ❏
The therapist and client identify the principal problem as tic or habit and understands key differences	Yes / No ❏ ❏
The therapist and client have distinguished clinically significant tics and habits from twitches and twiddles	Yes / No ❏ ❏
The client has learned to distinguish the tics from the habits; and these from other problems	Yes / No ❏ ❏
The client understands differential diagnosis between tics, habits, obsessions, twitches, and twiddles; client has filled in tic and OCD form	Yes / No ❏ ❏
The client has completed STOP and THAT and the therapist has discussed their importance with the client	Yes / No ❏ ❏
The client understands the rationale for the evaluation and that a good evaluation is an essential part of the program to apply the program effectively	Yes / No ❏ ❏
Client is suitable for the program based on assessment profiles: meets criteria for tics and habits; the tics or habits are clinically significant and cause dysfunction; does not have other problems requiring medical attention	Yes / No ❏ ❏

3

Motivation and Preparation for Change

In this chapter we consider client motivation by listing conveniences and inconveniences and discuss how to maintain client confidence in change. We look at: the reasons the client may wish to change and what the client will achieve without the tic and, in particular, client goals; how to reduce stigma and self-criticism and psycho-educate those around the client in adopting a helpful manner; using social support and the B.e.s.t. (Being there to Evaluate and Support your Tic progress) Buddy for encouragement; understanding that control comes more from acceptance of the tic or habit than fighting, replacing, or inhibiting it; and being aware of upstream and downstream dimensions of the context of tic or habit occurrence.

Motivation: Ready to Change the Habit

The client now has information on the tic or habit, and practice filling in the evaluation on the tic or habit, as well as identifying the problem and its severity and impact and identifying the style of planning and thinking. Ask the client for feedback and try to resolve problems with comprehension or form filling difficulties. This program is centered on the client and his or her habit. The steps and the rhythm can be individually tailored to the person's tic or habit, but it also depends on the person's motivation to achieve change. There is nothing mysterious about motivation. It does not mean having an iron will or boundless determination. Rather, motivation is facilitated by the following straightforward, easily graspable components.

Understanding the tic or habit—what makes an automated action into a habit?

The client's understanding of how to control processes leading up to the tic or habit such as thoughts, tensions, and reactions is essential to our program. The tic or habit itself is out of control once it occurs and the client may be misled by this fact into thinking that they cannot control onset. We define control as mastery of the processes preceding and leading up to the tic or habit, not resistance to the tic or habit itself, and more control may be achieved by doing less but

Managing Tic and Habit Disorders: A Cognitive Psychophysiological Approach with Acceptance Strategies, First Edition. Kieron P O'Connor, Marc E Lavoie, and Benjamin Schoendorff.
© 2017 John Wiley & Sons, Ltd. Published 2017 by John Wiley & Sons, Ltd.
Companion Website: www.wiley.com/go/oconnor/managingticandhabitdsorders

doing it more masterfully and economically. In the program we encourage reducing resistance and doing less.

Understanding it is possible to change

One of the advantages of our program is that we pinpoint the control the client already shows when not doing the tic or habit during certain activities and in certain contexts. The program identifies the strengths of the person and is often trying to build on these existing strengths to apply to more difficult contexts to broaden the client's repertoire. We do ask clients to act differently in contexts eliciting the tics or habits, but without requiring them to learn new skills or behavior; rather by extending existing competencies in their own repertoire, encouraging the person to apply the control over the tic or habit in low risk situations, and then applying the control to high risk situations. Change arrives bit by bit in following the steps of the program and never attempting a step the client is not ready for or capable of achieving. If we wish to climb a mountain via the steep face, it seems daunting but if we go by the circular path, it seems more achievable. The metaphors that we find most helpful are riding a bike, going on a long but picturesque hike, and, in particular, paddling effortlessly downstream past the stages of the program on a river. Client and therapist can use these metaphorical journeys to map progress (see client manual).

Feeling it is desirable to control the habit

We have to be clear on the reasons for the client's decision to change, and these must be positive. The inconvenience review lists advantages and disadvantages of the habit; it is important to keep these in mind throughout the program. However, it is also important that the person feels being tic- or habit-free allows more freedom to act as they wish, improves quality of life, but also allows movement toward goals and values, and achieving them in a more conscious fashion. So we ask the client to be clear on the goals of becoming non-tic or non-habit disordered. Obviously confidence builds as the client progresses along each step of the program, but certainly he or she must feel it is possible to change at the beginning and attain goals more easily. Please ask the client to fill in Table 3.8.

Surmounting obstacles

The client might encounter several obstacles en route that will impact on adherence. We have listed some, but not all, together with potential solutions, in Table 3.4. Obviously a high level of confidence, motivation, and understanding of the approach will help overcome obstacles. There is always a way around obstacles or roadblocks, as we call them, and the client and therapist just need some lateral thinking skills together with the help from the client's B.e.s.t. Buddy. We provide questionnaires on motivation and expectancy (see Tables 3.1 and 3.2).

Table 3.1 Expectancy therapy evaluation form (adapted from Devilly and Borkovec, 2000)

We would like you to indicate below how much you believe, right now, that the therapy you are receiving will help to reduce your problems. Belief usually has two aspects to it: (a) what one thinks will happen; and (b) what one feels will happen. Sometimes these are similar; sometimes they are different. Please answer the questions below. In the first set, answer in terms of what you think. In the second set, answer in terms of what you really and truly feel.

Set I

1. At this point, how logical does the therapy offered to you seem?

1	2	3	4	5	6	7	8	9
not logical at all			somewhat logical			very logical		

2. At this point, how successful do you think this treatment will be in reducing your symptoms?

1	2	3	4	5	6	7	8	9
not successful at all		somewhat successful			very successful			

3. By the end of the therapy period, how much improvement in your symptoms do you think will occur?

0%	10%	20%	30%	40%	50%	60%	70%	80%	90%	100%

Set II

For this set, close your eyes for a few moments and try to identify what you really *feel* about the therapy and its likely success. Then answer the following questions.

1. At this point, how much do you really feel that therapy will help you to reduce your symptoms?

1	2	3	4	5	6	7	8	9
not at all		somewhat			very much			

2. By the end of the therapy period, how much improvement in your symptoms do you really *feel* will occur?

0%	10%	20%	30%	40%	50%	60%	70%	80%	90%	100%

Table 3.2 Motivation questionnaire

	Yes	No
1. Are you seeking to change your tic for yourself?	____	____
2. Do you wish to please someone else?	____	____
3. Does your tic or habit cause you distress in your daily life?	____	____
4. Are there currently other major priorities to deal with in your life?	____	____
5. Will you be experiencing other major life changes in the very near future?	____	____
6. Do you understand and accept the rationale of the program so far?	____	____
7. Do you feel ready to commit yourself to regular practice of the exercises over 14 weeks?	____	____
8. Are you waiting for a magic pill to eliminate your tic?	____	____
9. Do you experience substantial benefits from ticking?	____	____
10. Do you believe that your tic is a permanent feature of yourself and that you will never get rid of it?	____	____

Changing the habit gradually and in a person-centered way

The program is cumulative, and progresses step by step at the client's pace, which is why we do not give fixed time points for progressing from stage to stage. It is important to master each stage before moving on. Mostly we are asking clients to do less not more and act naturally in accord with their natural repertoire. The program is paced so that the client will monitor improvements day by day. The principle here is errorless learning. Whatever happens during practice is a learning experience for the client, since, even if they don't complete the exercise, they will become more informed about the tic or habit and about how they cope with the tic or habit.

The therapist should always emphasize that this learning is advancing even if the client has difficulties and could not complete the exercises, since something has been learned from that challenge.

Realistic expectations of the program

In the meantime, we can provide the client with some realistic expectations of what benefits the program will bring if he or she follows the program closely. There is a good chance your tic or habit will improve. At least 70% of people following the program show clinically significant improvement and do not relapse. About 20% of these achieve complete remission and about 15% show no improvement. We are also good at identifying factors producing good outcomes and one is adherence to the program and practice of the exercises. The majority of people improve and maintain gains at follow-up. Some of the other reported gains include feeling:

- more socially confident;
- in control of muscles;
- able to move toward goals unhindered;
- calmer without the anticipation of ticking;
- less rushed because the client is less overactive and makes less redundant effort;
- more at ease in crowds because there is less need to suppress or disguise the tic or habit;
- less vigilant interpersonally;
- more able to adopt a calmer style of action;
- less attentive and less vigilant about the tic or habit and sensations;
- less worried about when the tic or habit will occur;
- able to eliminate strategies invested in disguising the tic or habit;
- Able to stop fighting with the tic or habit to suppress it.

Knowing how to stay on track

Staying on track means understanding and following the program in an orderly fashion and practicing the exercises as the person goes along. If there is difficulty the client and therapist can identify the stage where clients are stuck and discuss roadblocks. Redo the procedure or break it down into manageable, enjoyable small steps. The client can revise the exercises and diary daily to maintain confidence.

Self-confidence in controlling the habit

An important element here is self-confidence in the ability to change. Initial confidence in the client's self-control can be helped by:

- realistic expectations of achieving progress bit by bit over the course of the program;
- receiving feedback from your daily record and B.e.s.t. Buddy on progress so far;
- thinking positively about what clients have accomplished;
- always keeping in mind future goals and aims;
- adopting the correct metaphor of change (a trip down the river) to chart your progress (more on thinking and language later).

If you find that the client's confidence is flagging, you can ask:

1) Why is the client discouraged?
2) Is it a specific stage or technique? If so go back, redo and simplify.
3) If it is general discouragement, go over goals and inconveniences.
4) Recap all that the client has accomplished so far including existing control and discoveries of strengths.
5) If the roadblock concerns an exercise in the program, look at what the client is attempting and attempt less or clarify the exercise or take another route around the roadblock.

Maintaining confidence

It is important to maintain confidence in change throughout the program. Confidence builds with accomplishment, but it is an important motivator of change in itself. To keep up confidence it is important:

1) to receive constant feedback on achievements so far;
2) to think positively about progress and how far the person has moved along the path;
3) to go at the person's own pace—the exercises are cumulative but clients complete each one at an individual rhythm;
4) to think and act realistically and using SMART techniques (each step is Specific, Manageable, Achievable, Realistic, and has a Timeline);
5) to map progress on the chart and discuss with the B.e.s.t. Buddy;
6) to fill in the scale we have attached with the client every now and again to measure current level of self-confidence.

Confidence scale

No confidence in control (0)_____ _____Confidence in control (10)

Social support: Family, friends, or trusted other B.e.s.t. Buddy

Here, we discuss the difference between constructive or high quality or unconstructive or low quality social support, the importance of social support for quality of life, and different degrees of social support.

Table 3.3 B.e.s.t. Buddy form

Being there to evaluate and support the tic program

I _____ will undertake to encourage and support
_____ in his/her following the tic program including:

    Helping evaluate the tic.
    Commenting positively on progress
    Evaluating small steps
    Suggesting regular rewards
    Congratulating on completing the program

Name: _____
Signature: _____
Date: _____

Table 3.4 Roadblocks and solutions

Roadblocks	Solutions
No time/other priorities	Plan for priorities
Other problems could interfere	Discuss your engagement in program
People could interfere/no support	Make client aware of goals
Tic really not that important	Discuss ambivalence. Revise goals and inconvenience review
Receiving other treatment	Complete other treatments
I have gone so far but can't go any further	If client is stuck, discuss beliefs about progress

Social support can be at different levels but should always meet the criteria of constructive social support. Support from the client's friends and family can be very useful but it must be informative and constructive and not critical or judgmental (see close other and social support guide in Tables 3.5 and 3.6). Friends should encourage the client in their progress on the program and in completing the exercises, applaud even a small amount of progress, provide feedback on strong points, avoid criticizing the client for the habit, and reward the client for little successes. The client's *B.e.s.t. Buddy* is his or her "**B**eing there to **E**valuate and **S**upport your **T**ic progress" buddy, and is ideally a friend or relative or acquaintance in whom the client has trust and confidence, and who has the client's best interests at heart. We give criteria for high quality or low quality social support (see Table 3.5, 3.6) and on how to choose the client's B.e.s.t. Buddy in the client manual. The B.e.s.t. buddy is ideally someone the client trusts, someone honest, in whom the client has confidence, who understands the program, is willing to devote time and patience to helping the client in awareness exercises throughout all the steps of the program, and who will reward the client with encouragement every step of the way. In Table 3.3 we provide an outline of an agreement to be signed with the B.e.s.t. Buddy.

As we note later, a B.e.s.t. Buddy can also help monitor the client's tic or habit. Another person may notice patterns that the client misses, like breathing patterns, whole body movement, postures, and small expressions (see Table 3.3).

Table 3.5 Social support

Who?	Type
Husband/wife	Intimate
Family	Expressive
Friends	Acceptation
Acquaintances	Interactive
Organizations	Esteem

$$\text{Support} = \frac{\text{number of people} \times \text{diversity}}{\text{quality} + \text{satisfaction}}$$

Table 3.6 Quality of social support

High quality		Low quality
Being emotionally receptive	vs.	Criticizing/rejecting
Listen to the person speaking Example: How are you feeling? How was your day?		I don't want to hear you talk about your tic or habit disorder
Having a realistic perception Example: Yes you have a tic or habit disorder, but it is treatable, you have other positive traits		Dramatizing Example: Having a tic or habit disorder is terrible, it mean you have a mental sickness, you'll never be normal
Helping in a practical manner Example: How can we help you the best possible way?		Discouraging comments Example: No, stop, I'll do it, you can't do anything
Being a co-therapist Example: You are getting better gradually		You did it properly, but there is still a lot to deal with. Yes but. . . comments

Social support can take diverse forms and, assuming it is quality support, it will yield satisfaction regardless of type.

Different types or levels of support can be useful:

- The individual understands very well what the client is currently going through and can offer him or her constructive help.
- The individual understands a little about what the client is currently going through, but will try to learn more about it.
- The individual does not understand what the client is currently going through, but he or she is there for the client.
- The individual knows the client is currently having a hard time and can offer the client practical help.
- The individual does not need to be aware of the client's difficulties. He or she considers the client as someone who has value and interacts with him or her as he or she would interact with anyone else.

Tic and habit disorders are a problem and not a person.
Clients should be on their guard against the following:

- a tendency to identify with the tic or habit;
- acting and talking as if the tic or habit is an attribute;

- believing that the tic or habit can explain all behavior and problems;
- using the tic or habit as an excuse not to live fully;
- not recognizing other positive qualities;
- minimizing or rejecting positive comments;
- associating the tic or habit with parts of your personality;
- considering the tic or habit as part of your personality.

Rewards

The exercises are designed to be stimulating and engaging, but practice can be more fun with little rewards for practicing, planning in advance, and seeing through roadblocks. We have broken down exercises to a few minutes per day. In addition the client will receive regular feedback on his or her progress from their diary graphic and their B.e.s.t. Buddy or "Change Chum." A good way of planning a reward is to tell the client to give him or herself a treat every day, another one every week, and another every month, and after he or she has accomplished every step of the program. The rewards could be magazines, trips out, visits, or clothes.

Fix a weekly and monthly reward schedule with the client.

The Pros and Cons of Tics and Habits; and Setting Goals and How to Attain Them

It is important to be clear that seeking treatment is going to improve quality of life and functioning, and help achieve goals more smoothly. It is important that the client does not simply want to get rid of a negative habit, or that he or she is not seeking treatment for the benefit of someone else, whom the tic or habit irritates. The best motivator for changing a habit is moving toward a goal, not running away from unpleasantness.

It's important to keep a clear idea of what getting rid of the tic or habit will permit the client to be, to do, and feel. We ask the client to fill in the inconvenience review or pros and cons and goals; in other words, what they aspire to attain without the tics or habits, or the person they aspire to become. But we need to make this tangible in terms of what change means to the person. We have filled in some examples of inconveniences resulting from a tic or habit and positive reasons to follow the program. We've already established the desire to change the tic or habit and not to please others. The impact on others is important, but we also need to identify goals central to the person, so there is a goal to not ticking and the person is not simply escaping the tic or habit. The therapist can cover the conveniences and inconveniences of the tic in everyday life. At the same time this may raises questions about perceptions of the tic (see Tables 3.7 and Table 3.8).

Are there any conveniences you see to keeping your tic or habit? Perhaps you feel it makes you eccentric or it elicits sympathy? Be honest and ask yourself, are there any merits to having a tic or habit? Bringing any benefits out into the open will better enable you to evaluate your motivation to eliminate the tic or habit. You may also profit from asking yourself if these are really benefits or just facts you've learned to live with.

Table 3.7 Inconvenience review sheet

Please make a list here of all the inconveniences you have noted that the tic brings to your daily routine and of which you wish to be rid. These inconveniences can include avoidance of activities, fatigue from the tic or habit, and judgment of others or psychological effects, such as feeling odd.

Once you have made an exhaustive list of inconveniences, it is a good idea to reread it regularly to refresh your motivation and remind you of why you wish to eliminate your tic.

Inconveniences

Example: I avoid social settings

. . . .

. . . .

. . . .

. . . .

. . . .

. . . .

. . . .

Conveniences

Example: My tics make me appear to be a character

. . . .

. . . .

. . . .

. . . .

. . . .

. . . .

. . . .

. . . .

. . . .

Table 3.8 My goals

When I manage my tic, my goals are:
Examples: Partaking in sports
More at ease in social settings

If you feel strongly that your tic or habit is beneficial, clearly there may be little motivation to change it.

Client's Perception of the Tic or Habit

Before we change a habit we need to consider very carefully the pros and cons, because if we are to invest in changing it and complete all the exercises, we must be clear of the full impact on us of keeping or changing the habit. As an adult, chances are the tic or habit has become integrated into one's personality and its presence may just be accepted as part of life. The person can accommodate the tic or habit and just get used to living with it. It is important that the tic or habit be considered as a problem separate from identity. A phrase we frequently repeat with clients is that a tic or habit is a problem not a person. To help reflect on this point we include a one-item integration question to assess the degree to which the client believes the tic or habit is part of him or herself or not. One of the characteristics of tics or habits in adults is that they tend to be better integrated into the person's behavior. The person may even feel they are more of a character due to the tics or habits. There was a surgeon who achieved notoriety because he could suppress his tics or habits during surgery but let them go afterwards. However, if the clients list all the pros and cons of having tics or habits, they will generally find the cons outweigh the pros. This can often be because of unconscious avoidance of situations out of habit without even realizing it.

The client believes the tic or the habit is part of him or herself	Yes / No ❏ ❏
The client believes him or herself to be separate from the tic or the habit	Yes / No ❏ ❏
The client's motivation is assessed in terms of the understanding of the mechanics of change, desirability of change, and obstacles to change	Yes / No ❏ ❏
The client's self-confidence is evaluated and monitored, and questionnaires on motivation and expectancy have been completed	Yes / No ❏ ❏

Hidden hassles

As well as accommodating the tic or habit and becoming used to it as part of life, clients may also avoid situations and adopt habitual strategies to camouflage or disguise the tic or habit as a matter of course. We give a few examples below. List now in the space below all the situations the client avoids out of habit without realizing the restrictions.

- The client may avoid brightly lit settings.
- The client may avoid social settings, sports, or concerts.
- The client may avoid face-to-face meetings, preferring to communicate by telephone.
- The tic or habit and associated tension may cause difficulties in paying attention or carrying out tasks.

Tom, for example, had serious eye blinks, several hundred per minute. They were particularly pronounced when he was in social settings. So, in order to mask them, he would wear dark glasses. He eventually got a reputation for wearing his dark glasses like a rock star and it seemed to him he attracted attention. The downside was situations requiring observation and dark rooms where he had to take them off and had problems paying attention, and of course the blinks were obvious and fatigued his eyes. Tics or habits and associated tensions may prevent the client from paying full attention or carrying out and completing tasks adequately.

Situations that I avoid because of my tics or habits

_____
_____
_____
_____

Dealing with Stigma and Self-stigma

There is evidence that children with tics or habits are bullied at school, although there have been many advances in psycho-education amongst children and teachers (for further information, see Thibert, Day, & Sandor, 1995). In adults, largely the stigma is invisible. Often it may be self-inflicted, since people with tics or habits tend to be self-conscious. One exercise we ask people to perform is to walk around a mall and note all the strange sounds overheard, and then think of the tic or habit and where it would rate on a scale of 1–10 in disturbing others. Usually there are at least two or three people in the mall who rate highly on strange sounds and behavior.

From my observation in the mall, I noticed the following _____
_____ people making gestures and noises making inappropriate gestures on a rating scale from 1 (little)–10 (a lot)_____. _____
_____.

Most people have "twitches" and "twiddles," which is to say they sometimes make jerky, abrupt, twitchy movements, or play with objects or their hair, twiddling the object around their fingers. Generally other people rarely remark on isolated characteristics of another person. Rather they see the person as a whole in terms of their mannerisms and presentation. The client may be tuned in more to look for characteristics because of the tic or habit. On the other hand, if the person looks closely everybody has some faults: it is a part of being human. So, in their mind, features may be exaggerated.

People with tics or habits may feel others judge them as weak, incompetent, nervous, and untrustworthy. Unfortunately, in classic films shifty characters were often portrayed with some form of twitch, as well as an English accent! But that's dramatic license. We have included a scale that measures the client's perception of what others think of the tic or habit. If the client is self-conscious about a severe noticeable tic or habit, the therapist might like to prepare a short piece with the client on psycho-education to normalize the problem and present to others and the family (see client manual).

How to talk about the tic or habit

A large part of psycho-education is dispelling myths. The tic or habit is not a sign of nervousness, but rather that tension builds up in different muscles, and actually is a sign that the client is too active. Another important point is to connect with other people's own habits and fidgets and repetitive movements, since everybody has had twitches now and again. It helps when clients are talking about their tic or habit to compare it to other unwanted habits and the fact that we all have unwanted habits and that a lot of movements occur automatically. That's all it is: just a tension habit and reflex, which says nothing about the client as a person. Does the other person have unwanted habits? There are very few reflexes that don't require our body to set them up. Everybody has reflexes. Tics or habits result from tension, so is the tic or habit the real problem, or is it produced by whatever creates the underlying tension? With habits, it's easier to see on a dimension, since many people twiddle a clip or pull their hair. Tics or habits seem all or nothing, but tics or habits need tension, both psychological and muscular, and tension can be built up over time by thoughts and beliefs about actions leading to ways of using muscles. It has been known for some time that it is possible to experimentally induce involuntary movements, but one way to explain the nature of a tic or habit is that it is an extension of the tense–release cycle found in many habits to reduce tension.

The worst people for judging tics or habits are the people with tics or habits themselves. They may feel shame, embarrassment perhaps, starting in childhood, and we know particularly that children can be unkind. Ask the client to reply to the following items to evaluate the social impact of the tic or habit.

Because of the tics or habits:

I feel others judge me badly.	Yes / No ❏ ❏
I feel others judge me as incompetent.	Yes / No ❏ ❏
I feel socially isolated.	Yes / No ❏ ❏

I avoid social activities.	Yes / No ❏ ❏
I don't join in team sports.	Yes / No ❏ ❏
I often lose friends.	Yes / No ❏ ❏
I stay at home rather than going out to meet others.	Yes / No ❏ ❏

Thinking about tics and habits

The client has already filled in the THAT questionnaire as part of the evaluation, so will be aware of how thinking about tics or habits influences tic or habit onset.

We have already discussed briefly what are termed meta-cognitions (anticipation of and thinking about the tic or habit). We know that the client worrying about whether the tic or habit will appear and trying to suppress the tic or habit is likely to be counterproductive: anticipation can provoke tics and habits. One influence we have discovered is the way clients are thinking about their tic or habit, before and during the client's tic or habit. This can be anticipation or belief in the inevitability of the tic or habit, or about how the client will deal with it. One of the strategies we emphasize here is accepting the tic or habit and viewing it differently: not as an alien presence to be battled, but as a sign of high tension levels, and onset depends very much on how the client views and approaches situations. The tic or habit is not something that happens to the client but something that is produced by an overactive way of preparing.

Part of this psycho-education is teaching family and friends what to expect in the program: that it is gradual and the client will be advancing bit by bit. The B.e.s.t. Buddy can help here (see advice for B.e.s.t. Buddy plus for family).

Control: Micro- and Macro-control

Very few acts are under complete control. Basically, when we perform an act we have the big picture in mind, but we only have a vague idea of many of the finer micro-movements. Driving is a good example: although we are vigilant about what happens on the road and ready to take control at any minute, there are also a number of actions(changing gear, looking in the mirror, adjusting the steering wheel) of which we are basically barely conscious. Think of the number of acts the client performs every day without really thinking or more specifically being aware of: tying shoelaces, playing a musical instrument, smiling, shaking hands. Indeed, if we focus on these details too much we interrupt the flow.

Sometimes to attain overall control we need less micro-control, which seems contradictory. Also, when we set an act in motion, although we control onset, we can't always control consequences, and so it is with tics and habits. We need to accept the onset of the tic or habit simply because it uncontrollable when it appears, but the processes preceding the tic or habit and producing it can be controlled. Fighting or inhibiting the tic or habit is not a winning battle—a bit like blaming the ticket agent when the plane is late. The tic or habit is simply a messenger telling the client that his or her tension is out of control.

An important point is learning about control. We have tried to underline the importance of the right positive kind of control or mastery. There is fighting control, which is a negative type of control leading to more tension and stress, or there is subtle control, whereby the client deals with the larger processes leading up to the tic or habit. We have identified some of these already, including thoughts and tension, and we will explore more. Fighting control, suppressing, holding in, disguising, avoiding, and distracting may make matters worse. As we have already noted it's best to consider the tic or a habit as an end result of processes, of which clients are more or less conscious. Part of controlling any habit is to become more conscious of it. In the next section we discuss awareness exercises in more detail. But the client can try this out with a minor habit, such as playing with a paper clip, or an annoying habit. Such focusing of attention on it can slow it down or even impede it. Sometimes this can interrupt routines such as tying shoelaces or playing an instrument. Now paying attention to a habit is a little more complicated, but it is exactly by paying attention to an unwanted habit that we can interrupt and undo it. Afterwards when we've replaced it with a new habit we need to go back to viewing the big picture so that the new action goes smoothly.

Conscious control

In Figure 3.1, we have identified 2 dimensions important in control of tics or habits: awareness and choice. What is awareness? Awareness is becoming conscious. A controlled action has both choice and awareness. Automated routines may be performed through choice but outside of awareness (e.g. tying shoelaces). Tics tend to occur unaware and out of control and with habit disorders there may be awareness but lack of control. The aim is to increase the awareness and control in tics and habits. Figure 3.2 illustrates the interaction of continuity of action

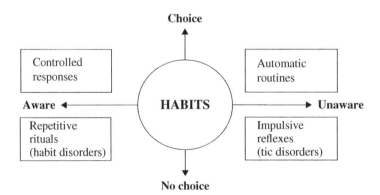

Figure 3.1 Reflexes, routines, rituals, and responses

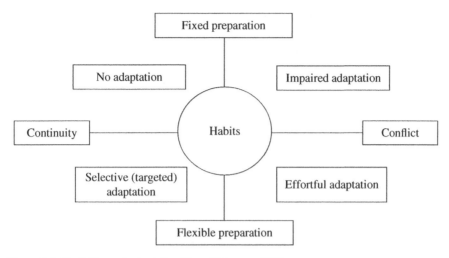

Figure 3.2 Flexibility and adaptation (from O'Connor, 2008)

and flexibility in planning. Being flexible with a continuous goal aids adaptation whereas a fixed or rigid preparation with conflicting goals impairs adaptation. But flexibility aids adaptation to conflict and if actions are continuous and flowing, adaptation may not necessary. But control begins with awareness and becoming aware can reduce superfluous effort to gain more flow. Mostly the client may have gotten on with life and ignored the tic or habit, thereby avoiding control rather than exerting it. Awareness brings the tic or habit into consciousness, and more consciousness means more positive control the client can have over the processes that matter and can be controlled. So control is double-edged: to exert control we need awareness of components, but on the other hand too much micro-control over small components means that we start to interfere with our actions. Full control or mastery means being confident in our actions and going with the flow without undue effort, conflict, and micro-control, and trying to direct the processes upstream that we can control and not the reflexes downstream that we cannot, leading us to a conflict type of control that impedes our flow and goal.

The Contextual Nature of Tic or Habit Onset

Now the positive bit. The client already has some control over his or her tic or habit, but he or she may not be aware of it due to contextual aspects of tics or habits. Tics or habits are worse or better in some situations and what influences this is a combination of elements—some surprising.

Ask the client: if you stop and think now, are there some situations where you are less likely to tic or habit than others, and we don't just mean when you are sleeping? These situations vary across people and are not uniform: for one person when they are stressed, another when relaxed. Often what defines a tic or habit-related or tic or habit-unrelated activity is the type of goal being pursued and to what extent the person is engaged or not. For example, a client of ours with severe whole body tics or habits suddenly ceased to tic or habit while immersed in playing the guitar.

Tics or habits are multidimensional and part of everyday actions. And, although it seems as though tics or habits occur in isolation, our whole body and environment are often involved, including our thoughts and beliefs. As we will see later in the program a consistent characteristic of tics or habits is that their appearance depends on situations and activities. Situations and activities where the tic or habit is less likely to occur or absent are important in realizing how habits vary, but can also be a revelation, as well as revealing strength. They illustrate situations or activities where the tic or habit is under some control—perhaps not consciously. Here, however, we place the emphasis on becoming aware and in particular recognizing downstream (other parts involved in the tic or habit besides the tic- or habit-affected muscle, such as thoughts, emotions, and behaviors at the time of ticking) as well as upstream factors preceding tic onset and becoming more aware of all aspects, physical, behavioral, thinking, both before and during the tic or habit.

In this chapter we have introduced crucial notions of how to approach controlling the tic or habit and how the program progressively addresses processes occurring at the same time and before the tic or habit. The next chapter covers getting to know the tic or habit. It is important to know how it appears, what form it takes, what muscles and other movement it involves, and also when it occurs and when it doesn't. As well as movements, feelings, moods, and thoughts can influence your tics or habits.

Therapist checklist for motivation

	Yes / No
Ensure that the client is ready for change and to follow the program	❏ ❏
Client's motivation is assessed in terms of the understanding of the mechanics of change, desirability of change, and obstacles to change	❏ ❏
Client's self-confidence is evaluated and monitored, and questionnaires on motivation and expectancy completed	❏ ❏
B.e.s.t. Buddy is identified. Agreement signed and the rewards schedule is planned	❏ ❏
Client has completed the inconvenience review, pros and cons of program addressed, and goals identified	❏ ❏
The client understands how to deal with stigma and how to talk about his or her tic or habit to others dispassionately	❏ ❏
The client grasps the difference between positive and negative control and how awareness and effort relate to control and to adaptation	❏ ❏

The client accepts they already have some control over the habit in low risk situations	Yes / No ❏ ❏
The client is aware of upstream and downstream processes contributing to tic onset	Yes / No ❏ ❏
The client understands how different ways of thinking about a tic can influence the tic or habit	Yes / No ❏ ❏
Social support is identified as a help in reducing tension and can be from diverse sources, but should be good quality support	Yes / No ❏ ❏

4

Developing Awareness

In this chapter we discuss how to identify the unit of the client's tic or habit of interest, defined around the principal tic or habit, and different methods to observe it and describe it; how to improve awareness and attention; and how to note premonitory urges and the principal parameters of the tic or habit, for example, by making a video and discovering thoughts, actions, and behaviors associated with the tic or habit using self-reflection and self-report. The daily diary helps in noticing how a tic or habit shows variation and in interpreting differences in the variation and understanding the wider implications of the contextual approach to managing tics and habits.

Choosing and Describing the Tic or Habit

How to choose a tic or habit unit

The client has listed all the tics or habits he or she is aware of in the previous evaluation section and, by filling in the forms, has identified his or her principal tics or habits and some physical and behavioral associations linked to the tics or habits. But now to implement the program in a targeted way we need to identify and manage the tics or habits one at a time.

So therapist and client can choose one tic or habit to focus on at the moment for the program, starting with what we will term from now on the "principal tic" or "principal habit." This is the tic or habit the person considers a priority because it is the most embarrassing, the most noticeable, the most annoying, the most dysfunctional, or for other reasons.

Description of chosen principal tic unit

_____

In addition it is important for the program that the tic or habit:

1) occurs at least once per day and is visible, and has done so for a year;
2) causes distress and the client is ready to work on it;
3) meets the criteria for a chronic tic or habit:
   a) has existed for at least 1 year;
   b) is frequent (at least one per day);
   c) causes the client (not someone else important) distress;

Managing Tic and Habit Disorders: A Cognitive Psychophysiological Approach with Acceptance Strategies, First Edition. Kieron P O'Connor, Marc E Lavoie, and Benjamin Schoendorff.
© 2017 John Wiley & Sons, Ltd. Published 2017 by John Wiley & Sons, Ltd.
Companion Website: www.wiley.com/go/oconnor/managingticandhabitdsorders

d) Is a priority to address for the person, and not someone else;

e) The chosen principal tic can be simple, complex, vocal, mental, etc. (see list);

The chosen habit can be any action that meets the habit disorder criteria (see Chapter 2).

This tic or habit will remain constant throughout the program and, should the client wish to change the focus to another tic or habit for whatever reason, they should continue to note the progress of this first principal tic or habit in addition to others. The client could list the tics or habits as, for example, my shoulder tic, my blinking, my hair pulling, and so on (Table 4.1).

How to describe the tic or habit unit

The next exercise is to focus in detail on the principal tic's form and nature. The client may have lived with a general idea or sensation associated with the tic or habit. But now we have to examine very closely what form the tic or habit takes, where and when it starts and ends, its components and their sequence, the muscles implicated, and, in particular, the background tension and bodily activity or posture from which the tic or habit arises and the accompanying breathing pattern. What does the tic or habit look like? In other words, what is the sequence of the contractions? What's its time course? Does it come in series? Is it accompanied by visible tensions? Which muscles are directly involved and contracted? Which muscles are indirectly involved (see Table 4.1 describing tic or habit)? Tics or habits can vary in form so we are interested also in the surrounding actions and behaviors that may vary with the tic or habit.

It is important to define the following characteristics: (a) the unit of the principal tic or habit, when it starts and when it ends; (b) what muscles and tensions

Table 4.1 Unit of tic description form

The sensations before, during, and after the tic, and all the muscles implicated before, during, and after the tic, need to be identified and described in the person's own words. This can be accomplished through studied awareness exercises or with the aid of a muscle movement detector (e.g., a lightly placed hand, a mirror, an electromyogram (EMG), or a video or external observer).

Tic identification

Tic: (in person's own words)

_____

_____

Muscles: behavior or muscle sequence:

_____

_____

Definition of unit (e.g., a full tic, a partial tic, or a sequence of tics):

_____

Any other characteristics:

_____

_____

are involved and in what order they occur—the client should pay attention to breathing at the time the tic or habit appears and pay attention to what other parts of the body are doing, particularly posture; (c) what activity was being undertaken when the tic or habit occurred, and what it was trying to achieve; and (d) attending to background activities—what else is the body doing, are there other thoughts on the backburner?

Awareness of the Tic or Habit

When we pay attention to something our awareness extends beyond the object itself. Awareness places our attention on a whole series of events going on around us. At any moment I might be concentrating on a particular arm movement, but my awareness of this movement includes the social, geographical, physical, and emotional context in which I am performing, as well as many other finer and more personal horizons and points of information. Now, some aspects of this awareness are themselves automatic, so I may be habituated to seeing and describing my habit in a certain way, say as a nuisance, a reflex, or have just "ignored it" or "accepted it." In other words, in some way or other, I have got used to living with the tic or habit problem. A first important step involves changing this habitual awareness. We discover the form and nature of the tic or habit by paying attention to it and going beyond the taken-for-granted assumptions.

Discovery of Seeing the Habit Differently

Paying attention is like any other ability and we get used to doing it in a certain way by focusing on some aspects and not others. The way to change awareness is by first and foremost changing the details habitually attended to in the tic or habit. But this change of focus requires developing the ability to concentrate on the tic or habit or tension whilst doing other activities—in other words dividing attention. When we perform an action habitually we pay attention to some parts but not to other parts. We want to widen this to observe other new points about the tic or habit. As a practice exercise ask the client to reach for something; now repeat the action focusing attention on how the foot moves. This is difficult—eespecially if the action is complex. It is difficult because it is difficult to divide up attention in a new way. Yet we divide up our attention all the time. It is just a question of habit. When we drive, we pay attention to different things at the same time. Dividing up attention in new ways is a question of practice, not capacity. In order to complete the next step of self-observation we ask the client to divide attention between two activities—the tic or habit and whatever else he or she is doing. Awareness performs an important function in controlling habits, since awareness can override automatic function, sometimes destructively, as when we focus on the single actions of doing up our shoelaces or playing the piano, but helpfully in stopping redundant habits like playing with a paper clip simply by becoming aware of them. Awareness by itself may inhibit twiddles (see Chapter 2) but not habit disorders.

A further point to remember is that awareness applies not just to details going on downstream at the same time as the tic or habit, elsewhere in the body, and the environment, but upstream to processes preceding the tic or habit, including thoughts about the tic or habit. Every seemingly involuntary process has a series of actions that puts it in place or sets it up. For example, the knee-jerk reflex only works when the client crosses one leg over another. This point applies to reflexes, neurological or startle, when a whole series of conditions needs to be in place for the tic or habit to occur.

A lot of the exercises are not only about discovering the nature of the tic or habit but are also practices in self-discovery, so in doing the exercises the client is finding out about the tic or habit but also about his or her own way of doing and being.

Discovery Exercises

There are three ways of improving the client's discovery:

1) By directly observing the tic or habit and behavioral and mental activity surrounding the tic with the help of the client's (a) B.e.s.t. Buddy, (b) a mirror, or (c) a video.
2) Through keeping a daily diary recording the elements the client has identified about his or her tic or habit (frequency, intensity, control, tension) covering the same time period (at least 1 hr) each day, and monitoring the client's thoughts and feelings as well as number and intensity of occurrences and control of the tic or habit.
3) Tracing the history of the tic or habit and identifying upstream processes, tensions, thoughts, and feelings that lead up to the tic or habit.

So the three tools to obtain feedback are:

1) Filming a video of the tic or habit.
2) Involving a friend or a trusted B.e.s.t. Buddy in observation.
3) Attentional focus by self-observation; monitoring via a mirror or another form of feedback; keeping a diary.

We recommend applying all three tools.

Making a Video: Replaying and Watching the Video

To film a video it is necessary to have a video camera or high resolution camera app on the client's phone and choose a situation where the tic or habit is likely to occur and can be produced in a camera situation. This may sound difficult but generally it's fairly easy to find with the client a situation or activity that triggers the tic or habit for the camera (we provide some examples from our experience in the next section "Advice for filming the video"). Habit disorders are more difficult because they are more easily suppressed. It may be acceptable to mimic the tic or habit action in a role play, but this should be a last resort if it is impossible to authentically reproduce a tic or habit trigger.

The client must also choose a situation where the tic or habit is unlikely to occur.

Obviously the video must capture the detailed contractions of the tic-or habit-affected muscle both during a high risk activity and, focusing on the same muscle, a low risk activity.

Advice for filming the video

1) Choose a situation or activity where the tic or habit is easily reproducible but likely to occur (e.g., boredom, writing, waiting, reading, listening).
2) Focus the camera on the tic or habit region and the muscles involved in the tic or habit.
3) Film for 10 min when the person is engaged in the activity.
4) Choose a situation or activity where the tic or habit is very unlikely to occur, which is reproducible for the camera (e.g., relaxing, playing an instrument).
5) Focus the camera on the tic or habit region and the muscles involved in the tic or habit.
6) Film for 10 min when the person is engaged in the activity.

Advice for watching and replaying the video

1) Try to watch the video with a friend, B.e.s.t. Buddy or therapist.
2) Replay the video several times at different speeds (particularly at slow speeds) if possible, noting different factors.
3) Remember the video is artificial in focusing on the tic or habit, which normally the client wouldn't do in everyday perception. Other people would not normally focus on an aspect but rather focus on the whole self. The client can be reassured as to the artificial nature of the video and its unusual focus on the tic or habit. Slow the video down to enable you to catch the beginning and end form of the tic or habit, and surrounding muscles and posture accompanying the tic or habit. Note from the video: the form of the tic or habit, the muscles implicated, the breathing pattern (does it occur on the in breath or the out breath?), the posture, the duration, and the intensity of other movements surrounding the tic or habit. Make observations on the posture and on other movements. Please ask the client's B.e.s.t. Buddy to fill in Table 4.2 after watching the video.

The client can be reassured as to the artificial nature of the video and its unusual focus on the tic or habit.

Involving your B.e.s.t. Buddy in observation of your tic or habit

Sit opposite each other and choose a situation or period likely to elicit the tic or habit. If necessary use the imagination to provoke the tics. In the event that the client cannot provoke the tic or habit, tell the client to mimic its automatic actions.

Table 4.2 Video monitoring form (the form can be copied and used also as a B.e.s.t. Buddy observations form)

Form: _____

Frequency: _____

Intensity: _____

Beginning: _____

End: _____

Muscle involved:	Respiration	Posture
_____	_____	_____
_____	_____	_____
_____	_____	_____
_____	_____	_____

Sequence of tic or habit (contractions in order of appearance):

1) _____

2) _____

3) _____

4) _____

Reaction to the video (often the client reacts to watching the video):

Examples: It's worse than I thought. Do I really look like that? _____

• _____

• _____

• _____

While the client is performing the tic or habit, his or her B.e.s.t. Buddy, without reacting to the tic, notes:

1) The muscles involved from the very beginning.
2) The sequence of the tic or habit: where it begins and ends.
3) Breathing pattern, posture, changes in posture, other visible tensions, other behavior.

Observation is made over several repetitions. If possible, especially with habit disorders, the action can be slowed down to capture all elements (Table 4.2).

Special considerations for mental and sensory tics

Here the client needs to describe the tic or sensation since it is not visible. The observer notes any accompanying changes in posture, breathing, or tension patterns. It is not possible to think without the body so there will be physical indices of the thinking tics.

Part of the observation is to trace the sequence of tic development. Perhaps the mental or sensory tic begins with a gesture, a subtle movement, a change in gaze or attention, or a hand gesture. Generally, the tic will have begun before the person first detects and becomes aware of it. This particularly applies to sensory tics. It is possible to experience the sensation in isolation but it may be the result of a previous tension or a sign of behavior to come rather than a stand-alone signal.

Premonitory Signs

We have covered observation of all factors occurring downstream in the client's body and thoughts at the time of ticking. Now what about the upstream dimension of processes preceding tic or habit onset? A controversial element is the premonitory urge. The premonitory urge is defined as a sensation or warning sign preceding the tic or habit that signals its arrival. This has been identified in a majority of tickers but not all and is measured by the Premonitory Urge in Tourette's Scale (PUTS) (Woods, Piacentini, Himle, & Chang, 2005). There is debate as to whether the premonitory urge is a sensation that appears to precede tension, a warning sign, or a sensory tic or habit in itself, or whether the urge develops with the tic or habit. We have included a questionnaire that details elements of the urge. We have added in thinking and feeling items in addition to sensations, since the premonitory urge seems mixed in with preparation for the tic or habit, which is active, rather than a passive sensation. The client may not experience the premonitory sensation, and that is fine. But it is especially important to pay attention to thoughts and emotions that precede the buildup. Is there a sequence? Is there a focus? What does the client detect as a warning sign before the tic or habit?

In the same way that we can break down the sequence of the tic or habit muscle contractions during tic or habit occurrence, we can do the same with the premonitory urge. When it occurs, what is the first thought or sensation the client notices that warns him or her that the tic or habit is imminent? Is it tension? Is the client expecting a tic or habit? Is he or she overvigilant to the body? What is the sensation?

The premonitory urge is complex and probably includes a mix of sensory signals, so we include here identifying components of premonitory urges and their timing and sequence of components. The premonitory components can include: sensations (e.g., tingling), tension (e.g., in the muscles), anticipation (or questioning if the tic or habit will appear), a vague fuzzy feeling, thinking of the tic or habit (e.g., vigilance), or being aware you could tic for some reason.

Evaluate the client's premonitory urge and note which components play a part (see Table 4.6).

An example of premonitory urge development in one client is given in Figure 4.1.

Specific examples for premonitory urges in the case of tics are given in Figure 4.2 and for habits in Figure 4.3. In particular, we ask the client to trace the sequence of what comes first in the premonitory sequence or timeline of upstream behavior to give an idea of the order of experienced phenomena leading up to the tic or habit (see Table 4.3).

The presence of components and their sequence will determine when the tic or habit begins and how these early components influence tension.

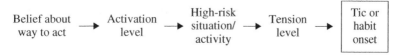

Figure 4.1 Model of processes preceding tic or habit onset

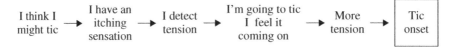

Figure 4.2 Model of processes preceding tic onset

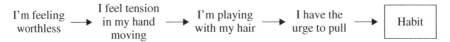

Figure 4.3 Model of processes preceding habit onset

Table 4.3 Premonitory signs

Please take note if the client experiences the following prior to tic onset:

- tingling warmth;
- tension: muscular or psychological;
- foreboding: feeling something will happen;
- anticipation;
- thinking about the tic;
- any other movement sensation.

Please note below the date and timing of the above and copy and keep as often as necessary to record the sequence.

Date	Timing	Premonitory signs
————	————	————————————————————
————	————	————————————————————
————	————	————————————————————
————	————	————————————————————
————	————	————————————————————

Daily Diary

Observing and recording the client's tic or habit

The first exercise with the diary is to keep count for 2 days of the number of times the movement occurs. If the tic or habit occurs infrequently, for example, only once a week, then extend the client's observation to 1 week. If there is trouble noting down or remembering, then it is best to make a mark on a sheet or card and tick off the response when it occurs as a line on a piece of paper, or use a counter.

The daily diary forms given in Tables 4.3–4.4 can be photocopied, and collated into a booklet. This booklet is compact enough that the clients can carry it and store it conveniently. We provide a prototype of the daily tic or habit diary and the characteristics to note in the diary. The client can practice for 2 days to familiarize him or herself with the procedure. We ask clients to keep the diary daily for 2 weeks before treatment starts and during treatment, and after treatment for a

Table 4.4 Daily diary

DAILY TIC DIARY

Your name: . . . .

Weekly diary dates: . . . . / . . . . / . . . . .To . . . . / . . . . / . . . .

Targeted tic: . . . .

Description: . . . .

. . . .

Tic unit is: . . . .

Tic recording period during the day is: . . . .

Abbreviation used in diary (e.g., for habitual situations/activities): . . . .

. . . .

. . . .

Other comments: . . . .

. . . .

. . . .

Date	Time	Frequency	Intensity (0–5)	Positive or negative control (−100 – +100)	Situation	Activity

(continued)

Table 4.4 (Continued)

Date	Time	Frequency	Intensity (0–5)	Positive or negative control (−100 – +100)	Situation	Activity

Note: To be completed every day for the specified time and tic for 3 months pre-treatment, during treatment, and post-treatment.

month for the same tic or habit unit and period. The therapist should consult the client's diary every week, reinforce the importance of keeping it, go over progress as reflected in the diary, and help construct a graph of progress.

Choosing a convenient time period of activity

The client can keep the diary for as long a period or as many periods as they are able each day. The minimum is usually 1 hr per day and we need enough time to capture the variation and to note how variation depends on activity. If the client decides to change tics or habits, this should be noted in the diary. Also, sometimes the movement comes in series and sometimes individually. If the tic is frequent then a shorter period may be sufficient. The unit will depend on the frequency of the tic or habit and whether it captures a representative enough period.

Another parameter to note is degree of control over the tic or habit. We noted in the previous chapter that there is positive and negative control. Negative control is fighting against the tic or habit, holding it in, suppressing it, and distracting oneself, disguising the tic or habit, or similar strategies that increase tension. The positive control strategies include eliminating or maintaining the thoughts and behavior that lead to tension, and generally accepting the tic or habit when it occurs, since it is an involuntary consequence of the tension buildup. In particular, mastery involves control early on of the way that the client plans action in an over-effortful and overactive way, which leads him or her to get caught up in planning and creating tension.

In the diary the client can note both methods of control, but can mark whether the control is positive or negative. At the beginning the client may be still using the tensing method of control, but as the client progresses the control will become more positive and the client will let go and relax the tension. We provide in Table 4.5 a guide to calibrate the scoring. Control is rated considering the client's

Table 4.5 Rating table for daily diary diagram

Frequency > 1 (per period)	Observable tics or sequences	_____
Intensity (0–5) (average over period)	Least intense—Most intense	_____
Control (0–5) (average over period)	No control—Full control	_____
Tension (0–5) (generally felt tension over period)	No tension—Extreme tension	_____

Calibration:	0 = Least ever experienced	Control:	0 = No control
	1 = Low		1 = 25% control
	2 = Low-medium		2 = 50% control
	3 =Medium-moderate		3 = 75% control
	4 = Strong		4 = 90% control
	5 = Strongest I have ever experienced		5 = 100% control

control over all the parameters (frequency, intensity, form) from 0–5: where 5 represents complete control in stopping the tic or habit; 0 represents no control, with the tic or habit occurring to completion; 1 represents an almost complete (75%) appearance; 2 represents a 60% appearance, wherein the tic or habit mostly occurred; 3 represents a 40% appearance wherein the client had some control; and 4 represents a 25% appearance of the tic or habit. Relative intensity is established by comparing the present tic or habit with the most intense episode the client can recall (5) and the least intense (0) (see Tables 4.4–4.8). There are other measures we take of the tic or habit as noted in Table 4.5.

1) The intensity of the tic or habit when it occurs; in other words its forcefulness.
2) The intensity of any sensations preceding or warning about the tic or habit.
3) The degree of tension as experienced during the tic or habit in the affected muscles.
4) Also, whether and to what degree the client considers they have control over the tic or habit and what strategies (positive or negative) are used to control the tic or habit.

The client can also note the urge to tic or perform the habit if the action is suppressed for any reason (Table 4.6).

Table 4.6 Measure of urge

Name: _____

Date: _____

How strong was your urge to pull out your hair/pick your skin/bite your nails/tics in the past 5–10 min?

1	2	3	4	5	6	7	8	9	10
Very Weak		Weak		Moderate		Strong			Very Strong

Table 4.7 Reactions to self-monitoring tic behavior

In what ways are you more aware of your tic?

....

....

....

Did you find the self-monitoring difficult?

....

....

....

Do you now feel more comfortable or less comfortable with your tic?

....

....

....

Are you better able to manage your tic because of the self-monitoring?

....

....

....

Has your attitude toward having your tic changed?

....

....

....

Did any aspects of the self-monitoring program require modification?

....

....

....

Has your tic increased? If so, explain:

....

....

....

The client may have difficulty at first in recognizing when the problem movement begins and the tension starts, which will have been helped by the video and B.e.s.t. Buddy observation, as these will have registered when the tic or habit commenced. This will become easier with practice, but for the moment the best strategy is to focus on the muscles most involved in the problem. Direct the client's attention to the large area of the muscle affected. As concentration on the muscle persists the client will discover that the focus becomes more and more sensitive and narrow, and the feeling for the movement and early detection of onset also sharpens. The client will not succeed in concentrating all the time, but, after a while, dividing attention between the initial movements of the habit will become well installed and won't require much concentration. After 2 days' practice the diary is now filled in daily and usually takes about 5 min to complete; consistently identifying the same tic or habit unit at the same time of day chosen with the client. Each week the therapist checks for completion and problems in completing, and recognizes and verbally reinforces the completion. If the person has trouble scoring the tic or habit since it is too frequent, he or she can score by sequence or make a rough estimate of the group or designated units of tic or habit occurrences.

Roadblocks to self-monitoring

Table 4.7 measures reactions to observing tics or habits, in order to allow the client to reflect on experiences and roadblocks; so let's foresee roadblocks the client may meet keeping the diary. *It takes too much time.* Actually it need not. Once the client has identified a tic or habit unit and a time completing the diary takes 5 min. *I can't be so accurate.* We realize the clients are using estimates. One roadblock that may discourage the client is that the tic or habit may seem to get worse, exactly because the client is becoming aware of the tic or habit. *I can't keep the diary because it reminds me of my tic, and keeping the diary makes it worse.* When we focus on any action, it tends to be highlighted, especially a body part. But this is not reality. *The diary makes me more self-conscious in public about my tics.* In reality people only notice big things, if they notice them at all. Most of those big things are personal, not physical. Also any augmentation of the tic or habit due to awareness is only temporary (Table 4.6).

Benefits

The benefits of keeping the diary are that it keeps the client aware of the tic or habit; it is mapping progress, which we can illustrate by drawing a graph of all the parameters with the client over a few weeks and seeing how the habit may have changed over time during the program; and it's valuable to see with the client if the individual measures change in synchrony or what measure changes first. This can be related to the client's experience; the graph of the scores over treatment monitors and gives feedback on progress. Clients sometimes forget their accomplishments and the diary entries can be a record of their success.

Tic or Habit Variations

Over the days of keeping a record of the tic or habit characteristics the client will notice the tic or habit varies and is more or less frequent or intense or under control on some days than others. Subsequently the client will become more aware of these variations and they are heightened when we develop consciousness of the habit and begin to systematically explore its variations. We are interested in noting situations where the tic or habit comes more or less frequently, where it varies in degree of intensity and degree of control even slightly. Identifying all of these is

Table 4.8 Summary form of variation over 1 week

Measure (intensity, frequency, control)	Degree of variation	Situations

essential to our management program. The client notes down all variations of the tic or habit in all parameters (intensity, frequency, control, and tension) and marks them down on the form we have provided in Table 4.8 over a period of 1 week.

Ask the client to monitor variation for a week so that the client covers a wide variety of situations. The client should try to identify situations where there is a high and low risk of the problem happening and try to be specific in completing this form. The client may, for example, record variations due to stress but he or she should be specific about what type of stress or what type of relaxing situations occur with the variation, and try to note down exactly what he or she is doing. For example, if it occurs watching television ask the client what activity is being undertaken when the problem arrives (e.g., watching a scary movie and feeling frightened whilst sitting on a sofa).

The therapist can encourage the client to realize that tics or habits emerge as a pattern in a context, depending on events preceding them and on underlying processes accompanying them.

The next step is to systemize these variations. Although labeling triggers in terms of large situations can be useful at the outset, we find it much more useful to look at activities since situations may be too general; for example, stressful or relaxing are general terms, whereas activities by definition are more active and particularly allow the client to identify what he or she is doing and thinking. A good way of defining an activity is to compare it with an alternative activity where the client does not tick. This brings out what is peculiar about the activity compared with other activities.

Tics or Habits in Context

Tics or habits always have a contextual profile; it's a defining characteristic, which means they are more likely to occur in some activities or situations than other. People with tics or habits rarely tic all the time and, if the client does perform the tic or habit all the time, it's pretty likely that it's not always with the same intensity. In fact a hallmark of tics is that it is possible to identify contexts in which they are likely to occur and contexts in which they rarely occur. This does not mean the tic or habit is completely absent in some contexts, but it may be less visible, frequent, or intense.

The other important point is to note downstream and upstream activity surrounding the tic or habit, which puts the accent on not only what is going on at the time of ticking but how the client approaches the situation prior to onset; that is, how the client anticipates, prepares for, and acts towards the situation. Indeed variation in activities can be accounted for by the different way people approach high risk situations before they tic or habit. This is helpful because even if the tic or habit is involuntary, we can control how we approach a situation, and hence indirectly we can control the tic or habit.

Why do we prefer the word "activities" to "situations"? Because ticking is an activity embedded in other activities. Tics or habits are motor phenomena, meaning they are actions. And although thoughts and emotions can influence actions, they tend to vary in what we do. Also, we did find that considering situations in isolation can be misleading, in that it may seem that a situation is associated with a tic or habit, but the physical situation may be associated with several behaviors. The client could be seemingly relaxed at home but mentally planning activities for tomorrow, for example.

Context plays a role in tic or habit onset probability, albeit in a highly idiosyncratic ways. Some people notice they are at higher risk of ticking in high arousal situations, for example, when engaged in a demanding task at work; some in low arousal situations, for example, when doing nothing at home. Anticipation of tics or habits may also increase the probability of ticking. Identifying which situations represent a high risk of tic or habit onset and which a low risk, and finding out what these situations may have in common is thus an important part of the functional analysis of tics or habits.

There are two complementary ways of accounting for this variation in tics or habits: functional analysis and contextual analysis. Both types of analysis are valid but explain different ways of viewing tic or habit maintenance.

It important to distinguish the idea of tics or habits as triggered by stimuli and hence performing a function in relation to the environment, and our idea that tics or habits are contextual and in fact are part of an action context and not necessarily independent or separate uniform responses triggered by different stimulus triggers. In other words, a stimulus or signal such as other people or the sight of a scab, in a stimulus–response sequence, can trigger the urge. We alluded in the introduction of Chapter 1 to theories that suggest tics or habits are triggered by environmental factors where they become learned associations. Both models are valid accounts of tic onset and relate to different levels of analysis. The tics or habits therefore serve a function and the person may receive a reward or a function through ticking. For example, a person ticking in a social situation may be ticking because they have learned to associate ticking with social situations, perhaps they have learned that it is acceptable or elicits sympathy and hence the tic or habit serves a function of some kind (see Figure 4.4).

Another way to view this is that tics or habits are contextual and vary as part of a context and are not independent uniform phenomena triggered by different triggers. In a contextual model, however, tics or habits are part of the cognitive psychophysiological activity in which they appear. Tics or habits are likely to vary in quality and form. They are an end point of the psychophysiological processes

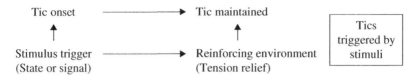

Figure 4.4 Functional approach

Figure 4.5
Contextual
approach

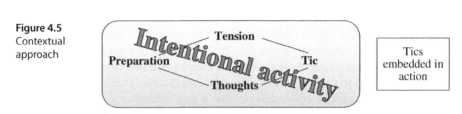

preceding them and hence we need to identify the processes which form part of the activity in which the tic or habit is embedded (see Figure 4.5).

The way in which the person approaches the situation, including their expectations, their intentions, their goals, and their posture flow, dictate tension leading up to the tic or habit onset. In the next chapter we systematize these contextual variations in terms of high and low risk situations/activities for tic onset and compare them to find the differences in how they are evaluated and approached.

Therapist checklist for describing the tic

Client identifies the single principal tic or habit unit or sequence according to criteria	Yes / No ❑ ❑
Recruitment of close other by client to help identify the form of the tic on the forms provided	Yes / No ❑ ❑
Recorded and watched the video and noted form of the tic	Yes / No ❑ ❑
Client has learned to pay attention to the tic and mastered self-observation of the parameters for the diary	Yes / No ❑ ❑
Client noted components of premonitory urges and their sequence	Yes / No ❑ ❑
Client kept the daily diary for 2 days and understood scoring of parameters in keeping the daily diary. Client willing to continuer to keep diary.	Yes / No ❑ ❑
Client understood and observed daily variation in tic parameters as shown in Table 4.7	Yes / No ❑ ❑
Client understands how tics can vary for functional and contextual reasons	Yes / No ❑ ❑

5

Identifying At-Risk Contexts

In this chapter we systematize the evaluation of the context around the client's tic or habit through identifying key high and low risk activities associated with tic or habit onset, and the thoughts and feeling that contribute to the activities. We also look more systematically at how the client evaluates the situations to arrive at an understanding of how the background to the client's tic or habit disorder.

Identifying Variations in the Context of the Tics or Habits

The client has already identified tensions, thoughts, behavior, breathing patterns, and postures that accompany tics or habits and precede them, either through video or observation, and also charted variations in intensity and frequency over 1 week and related them to an activity in Table 4.8. So, the client is aware that tics or habits show variations, but the variations depend on interaction between the client and the environment. So changing the environment can modify tic behavior, but we can also change context by changing our interactions with the environment. The environment is not an isolated stimulus, but a background that affords us certain actions depending on our projects, our actions, and our plans to act.

As well as discovering variations in keeping the daily diary the client may have noted both downstream and upstream processes associated with the tic or habit onset. Perhaps it was a discovery for the client to observe that not only do the intensity and frequency of the tic or habit vary at different times, but the form and behavior of the contraction associated with the tic or habit vary depending on context. When we are preoccupied with a problem there is a tendency to think that it occurs all the time. But as the client will have noticed the tic or habit appears or does not appear with some activities, whilst it is present in others.

Now the next step is formalizing these variations by rating their relevance to tic or habit onset.

Managing Tic and Habit Disorders: A Cognitive Psychophysiological Approach with Acceptance Strategies, First Edition. Kieron P O'Connor, Marc E Lavoie, and Benjamin Schoendorff.
© 2017 John Wiley & Sons, Ltd. Published 2017 by John Wiley & Sons, Ltd.
Companion Website: www.wiley.com/go/oconnor/managingticandhabitdsorders

Discovering High and Low Risk Situations or Activities

The client has noted tic variation over a fixed time period that represents a period during which the tic was likely to occur.

Now, it is extremely important to be precise and choose three situations/contexts in which the tic or habit occurs more frequently, and three contexts in which the tic or habit does not occur or occurs less. We are interested in what the client is doing; that is, the activity in these six contexts. In Table 5.1 we provide a template grid of what we term the high and low risk activities (activities during which the tic or habit is likely and unlikely to occur).

Here are some guidelines to choosing activities at high and low risk for ticking. The high risk activities should be activities during which the tic or habit is always likely or very likely to occur even though across high risk activities they may differ in intensity. The activities should be activities encountered regularly in everyday waking life. We need to choose three activities during which the tic or habit is most likely to be present and three activities during which it is less present or absent. If the client feels the tic is always present, then when we say absent we mean as minimal as possible in at least one tic or habit parameter (control, frequency, intensity, tension). We need three high and low risk activities as a kind of triple check on the motives and themes underlying the tic or habit, and three gives us enough examples to compare with each other and tease out similarities and differences in the evaluation of high and low risk activities It is important that the three high and three low risk activities are distinct from one another and unrelated. Also they can't be trivial (e.g., the client is asleep or deliberately inhibiting the tic or habit). The client might note, for example, that the tic or habit occurs less when he or she is working at the computer, so the client would describe his or her activity as precisely as possible. "Sitting with tension in arms and upper body focusing on the screen." Later on we will use the client's discovery of variation to be more specific about distinguishing processes preceding upstream from processes occurring during or after, and downstream context. An example is given in Table 5.1.

Table 5.1 Preliminary grid to extract high and low risk situations

Description of the situation (activity)	Level of tension (1–5)	Intensity (1–5)	Control (1–5; DNA)	Tic occurrence
Cooking	2–3	2	2	High risk
At work, in action	5	4	3	High risk
In the shower	1	1	4	Low risk
Doing exercise	1	1	3	Low risk
Doing cleaning (housework)	3	3	2	High risk
While eating	1	1	4	Low risk

Note: DNA = does not apply.

So the client can begin by noting down the situations and activities generally—again we have provided some examples to help. For example, the client might note "studying on my own," or "when I am in a social situation." This gives us the flavor of the situation but now, because the context is defined by the client's interaction, we need to know precisely what the person is doing. "Doing" here includes activity, feeling, and thought. Often when we are in a situation we are preparing for future events because there is always a wider context to our projects. So, for example, the client may be theoretically doing nothing watching the television but still mentally active and so may be subtly physically preparing to jump up and make a coffee in the kitchen. In this case the body reflects the two activities, watching the TV and preparing to make a coffee, with corresponding tensions. The activity should be noted rather than the situation. If it is easier, ask the client to first identify the situation then the activity in the situation. For example, the situation "in my car" becomes "in my car *driving to work*"; the situation "in the library" becomes "in the library *sitting and reading a book*"; the situation "in the kitchen" becomes "in the kitchen *cooking an omelette.*" The therapist's job here is to tease out the details.

Evaluating the Situation or Activity

The next step is to acquire more information on what typifies the client's evaluation of high and low risk situations or activities and what distinguishes them.

In Table 5.2 we have provided space for the client to arrange these three high and three low risk activities according to how likely the tic or habit is to arrive by ranking the three most and least likely according to the first bipolar dimension. (We provide an example of one client's experience pre-treatment and post-treatment in Tables 5.3 and 5.4. In the example, you and your client will note that post-treatment the ratings between high and low risk activities equalize. This illustration pinpoints an important part of the program, which is that it makes high and low risk situations more equal in terms of likelihood of tic or habit occurrence and activity evaluations.) The six activities can be scored on a scale of 1–7 depending on how likely the tic or habit is to appear during each activity. A score of 7 would be given if the tic is very likely to occur, and 1 if the tic is unlikely to occur. A rating of 7 indicates that the tic is almost certain to appear; 6 that it is likely to appear; 5 it is fairly likely to appear; 4 it may or may not appear; 3 it is fairly likely not to appear; 2 it is very likely not to appear; and 1 it is almost certain not to appear.

So the client lists the three high risk activities at the top of the three left hand columns and rates the activity 5–7 according to how likely the tic or habit is to occur. The client then lists the three low risk activities in the three spaces on top of the three right hand columns and rates how unlikely (1–3) the tic or habit is to occur.

Now the therapist and client can encapsulate the differences between these high and low risk activities in terms of how high and low risk activities are evaluated differently according to mutually exclusive bipolar dimensions (e.g., preparing to

Table 5.2 Grid for classifying activities likely and unlikely to be associated with tics or habits

	Situations/activities						
	High risk			Low risk			
	1	2	3	4	5	6	
Habit very unlikely							Habit very likely

Note: Identify situations at low risk and high risk of producing the tic or habit. Rank these situations 1–7 according to their degree of low or high risk of tic or habit occurrence.

Table 5.3 Pre-treatment example

	Situations/activities						
	Low risk			High risk			
	1	2	3	4	5	6	
	Cooking	Doing exercise	Eating	Driving	Writing notes (work)	Taking a walk	
Habit very unlikely	3	2	2	7	7	6	Habit very likely
Being healthy	3	2	4	5	4	4	Tired
Immobile	6	7	2	1	1	7	In movement
Pensive	5	4	3	5	5	2	Concentrated
Serene	3	2	4	6	6	4	Preoccupied
Confidence in myself	2	1	2	3	3	5	No confidence in myself
Comfortable	3	2	4	4	2	2	Afraid of being judged

Table 5.4 Post-treatment example

Situations/activities						
Low risk			**High risk**			
1	2	3	4	5	6	
Cooking	Doing exercise	Eating	Driving	Writing notes (work)	Taking a walk	
Habit very likely	2	1	1	2	2	1	Habit very unlikely
Being healthy	4	3	4	4	3	3	Tired
Immobile	6	7	2	1	3	7	In movement
Pensive	4	4	4	6	6	4	Concentrated
Serene	3	3	2	4	6	3	Preoccupied
Confidence in myself	2	2	1	4	3	1	Lack of confidence in myself
Comfortable	2	1	3	2	2	1	Afraid of being judged

be judged versus preparing to be at liberty). A good way to do this is to ask: "What is the difference in how I evaluate or experience situation/activity 1 compared with situation/activity 4, or between 1 and 2 compared with 5? Or I can compare 4 and 6 with 1?" There are a number of permutations for comparing one situation/activity with each of the others in order to elicit maximum dimensions of difference. Continue the dyadic or triadic comparison until the client has compared all high risk with all low risk situations/activities and decided in as many different ways as possible how the three high risk situations/activities are similar, what they have in common, and how they differ from low risk situations? There are 10 permutations for comparing high risk and low risk activities:

- 1 and 3 with 4;
- 1 and 2 with 4;
- 1 and 3 with 5;
- 1 and 2 with 5;
- 1 and 3 with 6;
- 1 and 2 with 6;
- 2 and 3 with 6
- 4 and 5 with 1, with 2, with 3;
- 4 and 6 with 1, 2, 3;
- 5 and 6 with 1, 2, 3. . .

The evaluations of high compared to low activities will tend to be mutually exclusive to the person. So if the high risk activities may all be activities in which the person feels judged: the low risk activities, despite being different activities, will tend to share the opposite characteristic of feeling free to express oneself. The evaluations associated with the low risk activities are scored 1–3 and the opposite evaluations associated with high risk activities are scored 5–7. So here there is a bipolar dimension between feeling judged (7) to feeling free to express oneself (1), with each high and low risk activity representing different degrees of either end of the dimension. So those activities where the client is feeling judged would be ranked from 5–7 and those activities considered free ranked 1–3. On the same scale (1–7) used previously to rate situations/activities according to whether the tic or habit is likely or unlikely to occur.

In eliciting evaluations differentiating the high and low risk activities we try to avoid large labels such as: "feeling good" versus "feeling bad." If the person uses an abstract or general evaluation, ideally this term can be made more specific. For example, if the person writes "tired" versus "on form" as an evaluation, this could be conceptualized as: "in this activity I'm worn out" versus "in this activity I feel fresh."

This comparing will require a little bit of thought, but it gives us insight into specific and subtle differences between these contexts in terms of the way the client thinks, acts, and feels, and also gives insight into his or her repertoire of how he or she constructs and evaluates his or her world relevant to tension and ticking. There are enough subtle combinations of comparisons to elicit quite a few personal themes, and the comparisons can be extended until a number of dimensions are elicited and the comparisons are exhausted. When the client has finished, there should be a figure from 1–7 under each of the six high and low risk situations/activities representing how each high and low risk activity ranks on each end of the bipolar evaluations elicited and depending on which end of the bipolar dimension is more likely to be present in the activity. So if the client is very bored during cooking he or she will put 7, but if he or she is not totally bored during cooking he/she will put between 1 and 7 in the space in the grid under each of the individual six activities. Any new evaluation dimensions can be added to the columns after the other dimensions elicited from the client and the presence of each end of the dimension scored from 1–7 for each of the six situations/activities.

Continue comparing two high risk activities with a low risk activity and vice versa until the client has exhausted all possible differences in how he or she evaluates high and low risk activities.

When the client has ranked to what extent his or her idiosyncratic dimensions apply to each of the high and low risk activities by rating them 1 to 7 according to how much each end of the evaluation applies to each situation. Now take the activity rankings along the first dimension (tic or habit likely or not likely) and compare them in turn to the activity rankings on each of the other dimensions for all six situation/activities. These rankings can then be matched with the rankings of how likely or unlikely the tic is to occur to determine whether the evaluation dimension is relevant to the tic or habit. If the score on the tic or habit likely dimension in each of the three situations is 5, 6, or 7, and the score of one end of the evaluation dimensions on these same situations is 5, 6, or 7, the evaluation dimension could be relevant to the tic or habit occurrence. If the score of the evaluation dimension is 2, 3, or 5 on the other hand, the evaluation dimension is probably not relevant.

The relevance of dimensions can be confirmed with the client. Depending on how the client evaluates the difference between activities, one end of the evaluation dimension may apply more to high risk and the other to low risk activities. The client can then see which each end of his or her evaluation dimension applies to each high and low risk situation.

In the example given, this comparison between dimensions reveals cooking as a high risk activity relevant to tic or habit onset and the evaluation dimension mobile–immobile seems the most relevant dimension, according to the scores given to each activity on this dimension.

The evaluations are idiosyncratic, and in our workshop exercises we found that no two people evaluate the same activities in the same way. The strength of this technique is that the opposite evaluations which are respectively relevant to high and low risk situations are not just opposite evaluations but mutually exclusive. The bipolar evaluations distinguishing high and low risk situations are not necessarily logical opposites (calm–stressed) but personal opposites (e.g., feeling judged vs. feeling free). This also gives a lever for recognizing the mutually exclusive contexts are associated with activities of high and low risks of tic and habit onset.

The discovery of how he or she valuated low and high risk situations differently and the strengths that the person already possesses in low risk non-tic situations.

Linking High Risk Activities and Evaluations to Feelings and Thoughts and Assumptions

Take all the evaluation dimensions which are relevant to likelihood of tic or habit, put them together, and ask the client what insight they give about the way he or she thinks, feels, or behaves during the movement problem. For example, if the dimension "with other people" and "unsure of myself" is important, ask the client to try to think of the thoughts that would come before he or she entered these situations, how these anticipations would translate into feelings about the self, and how this might lead to certain muscle tensions and postures.

The activities have specified the behavior and the evaluations naturally elicit feelings, but with knowledge of the feelings one can elicit the thoughts accompanying the feeling. As in:

"So you evaluate this situation as enjoyable?"
"Yes."
"Okay, what's the feeling associated with this activity?"
"I'm feeling engaged and happy."
"And the thinking?"
"I'm thinking I'm going to have a good time."
"You evaluated this situation as unpleasant, so what is the feeling associated with this activity?"
"I'm feeling bored and dissatisfied."
"And the thinking that goes with it?"
"I'm thinking I want to get out of here."

We talk later about how we get hooked on thoughts and behaviors that seem to predict the outcome of a situation but trap us with their inevitability.

Table 5.5 Linking thoughts, emotion, and behavior in high risk situations

	Thoughts/ Anticipations	Emotions	Corporal activity
Situation 4 Working at the computer	- I must augment my level of attention, I must focus - I prepare myself to give an intellectual effort -I tell myself that I must realize some certain work in a given time (deadline)	- Most of the time, a certain level of stress, or at least a tension, linked with my performance and/or my deadline - Generally, I feel positively motivated when I think of the results (positive stress)	- Body generally immobile, except hands - Seated, posture relatively straight - A little tense to very tense - Sometimes, with the fatigue and tension, breathing is more difficult
Situation 5 Talking on the phone	- Focused on the reason for the call, mental preparation (structure content) - In certain contexts, a certain apprehension	- Sometimes a certain level of "stress" - Personal call; feeling of relaxation	- At work, seated, but my hands are always busy (playing with work supplies) - At work, same thing or in movement doing another activity (e.g., dishes)
Situation 6 Planning	- I prepare myself to augment my level of attention, to concentrate/focus - I prepare myself to give an intellectual effort	- Sometime a certain apprehension - Other times, this activity calms me (when faced with what will be coming, what I will have to do)	- Generally seated and immobile, but sometime standing up - Posture relatively straight

In Table 5.5 we illustrate again how thoughts, tension, and mood are linked, and we ask the client to note down the thoughts, feelings, and specific muscle sensations associated with each high risk activity using the dimensions he has rated most relevant to the client's problem. Now that we have seen how tics or habits fit into windows of activity and constructs of situations, we can look further back at beliefs that influence our construing. So there is one more thinking element to our detective work. This is where Table 5.3 is valuable, since by comparing high and low risk activities, we establish themes necessary to define both, and from these themes we can specify the thoughts, feelings, and assumptions behind the evaluation.

Thoughts associated with the tic or habit evaluations deserve special consideration. In the next exercise we look at the link between the evaluations and thoughts and feelings occurring in the context of ticking (Table 5.6). So for example, if the client evaluated his or her mood during the high risk activity as being bored, possibly the thoughts associated are that "I am wasting my time here," coupled with a feeling of impatience. Thoughts fall into two groups: immediate anticipations of what will happen in future situations, during which the client

Table 5.6 Tracing beliefs from feelings and activities

Tic/habit/ activity	Evaluation/ experiences	Anticipations	Assumptions	Beliefs
Example: Reading a technical book	Frustration/ boredom	I won't understand	Technical books are difficult	I'm not very competent

may anticipate ticking or being awkward in front of others; or background assumptions, which may set up the anticipations about the situation. For example, an anticipation such as "I will not be at ease in a social setting" may stem from the assumption that other people will judge one. The difference between anticipations and assumptions is that assumptions tend to be more permanent and about general outcomes. Anticipations are immediate, short-lived, and punctual. But of course they can be linked and assumptions can encourage anticipations. Behind assumptions there may be long standing beliefs that can produce assumptions; in particular, beliefs about the client's appearance and the right way to act. If the client has these underlying beliefs it may be impeding progress, holding him or her up in adapting his/her approach. Ironically, changing the behavior side of tics or habits is more straightforward than the thinking side, since there are fewer beliefs and more habits. But beliefs are simply entrenched thought habits and can be modified by testing out their flexibility. We suggest the client notes down his/her assumptions and examines whether they are really valid, or whether they are too rigid and would benefit from flexibility in the light of the discoveries.

1) Watch out for assumptions by tracing them back from anticipations about situations and activities.
2) Note them down and note how they influence the client's behavior.
3) Do they really help the client along?
4) Are they flexible or rigid?
5) Are they useful and adaptive?
6) What would be the effect of changing assumptions and letting them go, on approach, feeling, tension, involuntary contraction, and preparation?

When the client has completed the form in Table 5.6, tracing thoughts about tics or habits, the beliefs given in the examples can be tied up in Table 5.7 with the constructs elicited from the evaluations of the situations in Tables 5.2–5.3. As the client will see, background beliefs and assumptions synchronize with the evaluations of high risk situations and dictate approaches to these situations.

Table 5.7 Anticipations, assumptions, and beliefs about actions or situations linked to tics or habits

Anticipations	Assumptions	Beliefs	Link to evaluation in grid
I always tic in social situations	Social situations are judgmental	People can judge me badly	Being judged vs. feeling free
I need to pay attention all the time	I can't move when attending	Tension means staying alert	Feeling tense vs. not stressed

Putting all this together we can see how behind high and low risk activities there are ways of behaving, thinking, feeling, and planning that can sometimes be traced back to anticipations reflecting rigid assumptions and firmly held beliefs. So now we can discuss introducing flexibility into thoughts as well as muscles in changing our actions.

Therapist checklist for contextual variation

The client identifies high and low risk activities or situations on the basis of the diary	Yes / No ❏ ❏
The client fills in the situations above the columns in the grid and rates them according to the presence of tics on the first dimension (1–7)	Yes / No ❏ ❏
The client is able to elicit bipolar evaluations by comparing the differences in experience between all high and low risk situations/activities	Yes / No ❏ ❏
The client links anticipations to inflexible background assumptions and beliefs	Yes / No ❏ ❏
Client links thoughts emotions and behavior associated with high risk situations (Table 5.5)	Yes / No ❏ ❏
Client compares permutation of high and low risk situations to elicit dimensions of evaluation separating high and low risk	Yes / No ❏ ❏
Ends of the dimension are labeled idiosyncratically and rated according to which end applies to each end of the dimension	Yes / No ❏ ❏
The ranking of the evaluations are compared to the tic likely dimension to see if evaluations are relevant to tic onset	Yes / No ❏ ❏
Client traces anticipations, assumptions, and beliefs linked to evaluation dimensions and high risk situations	Yes / No ❏ ❏

6

Reducing Tension

A key component of the program is introducing flexibility: both psychologically and physically. We plan to address physical tension practically, but even physical tension has physiological, behavioral, thinking, and emotional components.

In this chapter we cover how common actions, patterns of use, and postures can encourage tension. These include the way we prepare for action and how we regulate tension. In this section we will learn to become more aware of tension. The client will discover:

1) The link between movement posture and tension.
2) How to use muscles efficiently and isolate actions.
3) How to gain more flexibility in movement.
4) How to gain more control of muscle reactions.
5) How to avoid creating conflicts and frustration.
6) How to give more flow to his or her actions through harmonizing movements with goals and values.
7) The importance of the dimensions of style of preparing for action.

Tension Before Ticking: How to Use Your Muscles

Muscles, of course, do the work of the body, but they also in turn work the body. Figure 6.1 is a schematic diagram of the reciprocal relationship between muscle output and feedback and feed forward to the brain. An important task of the muscles is their feedback function, which not only gives the brain information on location and orientation of the body, but also influences expression of emotion. The flow of movement depends as much on the state and flexibility of the muscle as on the coherence of the action plan. In other words, how the client plans action influences the way the muscles prepare for the action, and, together with how the client interprets feedback of the action, these are all equally important for any movement to progress smoothly. Equally important is the feed forward function, which allows us to plan and prepare the muscles for action to come.

Following the diagram in Figure 6.1, the client might like to test out and experiment with recognizing muscle use by enacting a fast, a slow, and a hesitant movement. Muscles, like people, can be in a variety of states—they can be relaxed or

Managing Tic and Habit Disorders: A Cognitive Psychophysiological Approach with Acceptance Strategies, First Edition. Kieron P O'Connor, Marc E Lavoie, and Benjamin Schoendorff.
© 2017 John Wiley & Sons, Ltd. Published 2017 by John Wiley & Sons, Ltd.
Companion Website: www.wiley.com/go/oconnor/managingticandhabitdsorders

The elements in the boxes determine how the brain and muscles respond

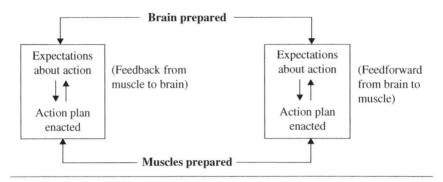

Figure 6.1 Flow of movement organization

inflexible, ready or unready, efficient or inefficient. Muscles are sensitive instruments, responsive to even a slight change in intention on the client's part. In addition, they are always part of a target pattern or profile of action. This is why it is difficult to ascribe a function to any one muscle in isolation, since in performing any task a series of muscles will inevitably be involved; several muscles play a supportive role even if they don't move. In Table 6.1, we list a number of muscles involved in selected everyday functional actions.

In Table 6.1, we note muscles principally and functionally involved in common actions. But people with tics and habits typically invest effort in redundant muscles as in, for example, contracting the face muscles at the same time as blinking instead of just the eyelids. Ask the client if the distribution of energy is appropriate

Table 6.1 Everyday actions and principal muscles involved

Standing up:	Tension in legs, abdomen, buttocks
Sitting down:	Lean body forward and tense thighs, buttocks, and abdomen until body lowered or lifted and back is straightened
Walking:	Tension in feet, legs, and arm swing. Peel foot off the ground and pass over ankle of other foot, swing arms in opposite direction to leg
Talking:	Face, eyes, mouth, and hand gestures
Holding a telephone, or knife and fork:	Tension in hand only
Picking up a suitcase /carrying shopping:	Bend knees, tension in arm and shoulders and stomach
Typing/writing:	Tension in fingers, and involved hand and eyes
Watching TV:	Eyes
Sitting still doing nothing:	No noticeable surplus tension anywhere

when performing these actions. Is there tension in parts that do not contribute to the action? Is the client over-tensing in a muscle or muscle group? For example, does the client over-tense the biceps when throwing a switch? Does the face tense up when lifting up a suitcase? Some of this superfluous action may relate to the degree of anticipation or preparation that the client is investing in the action. This goes back to what we said earlier about the brain and body being related. Because the body must prepare for the future and the future is unknown, anticipation comes into play. We might be using the same arm action to flick a switch as to open a door, or putting on a summer jacket in the same way we'd put on a winter anorak, or preparing to address a crowd when we are talking to a single person. Compare the client responses in similar tasks that require more or less energy and see if the client is adequately discriminating between them in terms of muscle use and efficiently distributing energy and tension. Sometimes, we automatically use the same muscle for a heavy task after performing a high task.

Part of becoming more flexible in the use of muscles is to discriminate and to localize actions to the correct muscles and not involve redundant muscles. One problem we have noted is that tension can often be produced by activating non-relevant muscles; for example, tensing the face when lifting a glass. This redundant tension may be because the client is preparing for more than one action or a tension adopted through habit. The problem is that because this redundant tension is not useful it does not adapt but hangs around as tension; for example, if the client lifts up a suitcase with his or her arm muscle the muscle will adapt to the weight. But if the client's face muscles tense up, this tension is redundant to the lifting and, since it is not functional, it will not adapt to the lifting. *We don't want superfluous tension.* The client could practice with the therapist and at home in performing certain actions including high risk actions to see if he or she uses redundant muscles referring to the list of efficient actions and muscle use in Figure 6.1. The client can improve movement coordination and flexibility by doing physical exercises, or by enrolling in courses concerned specifically with changing quality of movement and coordination and posture such as tai chi, mime, Feldenkrais, Alexander technique, qigong, or yoga meditation. Movements are the most adaptable aspect of behavior, and there is no dimension of movement flexibility, flow, coordination, speed, or deliberation that the client cannot train differently, whatever the client's age or limitation on the client's movement. All flexibility requires is awareness, an open attitude, and practice (see Table 6.2).

Ask the client to try an exercise now. Ask him or her to try reaching to pick up a pen and to slow down the action to capture the movement. What muscles does it involve? What muscles does the client need to activate to pick up a pen? Forearm, eyes, fingers? What muscles does the client not need to activate? Face, jaw, other arm, legs? Is there a difference if the client reaches out blindly for the pen or if the client plans ahead for the position of the pen? Also, is the movement easier if the client carries it out placing the pen with one aim in view or with mixed or uncertain aims? "I'll place the pen here or maybe there or perhaps not." The client can note how smooth or staccato is the style of action when under ambivalent or directed action. In order to capture the influence of preparing two conflicting tasks, the client can try to reach and to inhibit reaching at the same

Table 6.2 Flexibility exercises

When the client is performing everyday actions, is the client investing too much effort? Are parts of the client's body doing jobs they need not do? Is the client's face or tongue helping the client lift up a suitcase? Are the client's legs helping his or her hand write a letter? Are the client's shoulders helping his or her eyes read a book?

The following are more active exercises to test the client's economy of movement.

1) Ask the client to stop an action, such as getting out of a chair or writing, and freeze in a time frame. Then monitor all the tensions present in the client's body. Are they all relevant to the task?

2) Ask the client to imagine him or herself about to perform an action and see which muscles spontaneously tense up.

3) Ask the client to perform an action under time pressure and without time pressure to see the difference in tension level.

4) Ask him or her to deliberately tense non-relevant muscles in an action to see the difference in performance compared to when these non-relevant muscles are relaxed.

5) Ask the client to perform an action that is usually automated, such as knitting, playing the piano, tying up his or her shoelace, and then stop midway and focus on each element of the task to make it a more controlled action. How does this affect the performance and the feeling?

6) Ask the client to try preparing to do two different tasks when normally he or she would only plan for one; for example, writing with a pen, but also holding it as firmly as possible. What effect is there on performance?

time and notice how jerky and paralyzing the movement becomes when trying to do two opposing tasks.

Ask the client to try another exercise: supposing he or she sets about the task of trying to accomplish three tasks inside 10 min. Let's say the client decides to reply to emails, write a letter, and listen to the radio. While trying to accomplish all these tasks, what happens? Well, the client may switch from one to another, but the mind is never fully on one task and, most of all, the client doesn't accomplish them all. Now ask the client to try to carry out two tasks. Does s\he notice the difference compared with trying to achieve multiple differences? Is it more feasible? Is the client more focused? Is the client calmer? Does the client feel more in control? Now ask the client to try doing just one task. There are two ways of interfering with smooth action: trying to do too many tasks at the same time, or making too much effort in carrying out an individual task. Which way produces more tension? Which produces more satisfaction? Which way allows more focus on the here and now?

Tension is not a state that just arrives but is rather a state produced by our muscle use, in particular reacting and preparing for action. Here are some guaranteed ways of producing chronic tension:

1) Consistent overuse of muscles.
2) Habitual overpreparation, overinvestment, and overeffort in activity.
3) Constantly preparing for an uncertain event.
4) Always trying to do too much at once.

5) Preparing for one action but doing another at the same time all the time.
6) Making preparation to carry out two incompatible tasks (see Figure 6.2) pushing and pulling the client in different directions or even opposite directions.
7) Insisting on being in advance of oneself and planning for the next task while
   still engaged in the present one.

People with tics or habit disorders tend to have higher levels of tension which
can be monitored. Ask the client to fill in the Tension scale in Table 6.3.

Another relevant factor to do with effort is how the client decides that an
action is accomplished. Is it based on the feeling that the client has expended
effort rather than on the perception that the task has been accomplished? Often
people with tics and habits rely on how they feel to decide whether they have
performed enough or correctly rather than just relying on visuo-spatial cues.
Relying on the feel is an inaccurate way of gauging accomplishment since the
feedback is "feels good" or "just right," which is a subjective measure of effort
rather than a visible sign of completion. Sometimes people will rely on both but
nonetheless not be satisfied unless the feel is right. Relying on tensions, as we
have noted, often leads to performing conflicting tasks either within the same
task or performing two jobs at the same time in order to get feedback from the
effort. The two tasks are competing for resources and slowing the client down,
pulling the client in different directions, making the client inefficient and leading
to frustration.

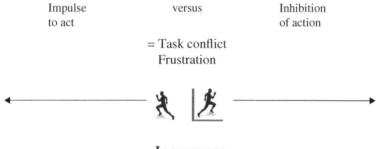

| Impulse | versus | Inhibition |
| to act | | of action |

= Task conflict
Frustration

In summary

A conflict between inhibition and impulsivity leaves the individual trapped in a
frustration–action cycle, and he or she cannot move forward with a goal-directed behavior

Example

INHIBITION	IMPULSIVITY
On the phone with a friend	Behind on daily tasks
Trying to be polite and make a good impression	Want to end phone conversation

Figure 6.2 Frustration–action cycle

Table 6.3 Tension scale

	True	False
1) I always feel tense	_____	_____
2) I feel tenser in some muscles than in others	_____	_____
3) Whenever I perform an activity, I feel a tension in parts of my body	_____	_____
4) I am unable to relax completely	_____	_____
5) I am aware that I tense unnecessarily when I perform an action	_____	_____
6) Others have remarked that I look tense	_____	_____
7) My tension is causing me other problems, like pain and immobility	_____	_____
8) Even thinking of an activity or event can increase my tension level	_____	_____
9) The tension drains my energy	_____	_____
10) I don't seem to be able to live without tension	_____	_____
11) I restrain my activities due to my tension	_____	_____
12) It's not possible for me to function without tension	_____	_____

Conflicting Preparation Versus Coherent Preparation

One way of not preparing efficiently to carry out a task is to prepare for two incompatible or competing tasks at the same time. This may involve contracting redundant muscles, inhibiting or distracting the client from his or her action and generating conflict. Ask the client to try writing as neatly as possible while holding the pen as tightly as possible. Ask him or her to try to carry out any fine motor action whilst maintaining a high degree of tension. Ask him or her to try to move forward and hold him or herself back at the same time. Much over-preparation and overinvolvement is explainable by spreading activation and association of non-pertinent elements: where a particular reaction or activation spreads to non-relevant or unnecessary muscles or functions.

So let's take John's shoulder tic or habit. If we asked John about his tic or habit, he would say it was in the shoulder. But when we look at it closely we find that it actually involves the arm and the chest, so both move at the same time as the shoulder together on an in breath. In addition, there is an in breath and the tic or habit is worse when he is sitting, unoccupied. So what does John do when the tic or habit occurs? He tries to hold it back, suppress it, or disguise it. He also is deeply embarrassed by it. In fact, although not aware of all the ins and outs of his tic or habit, he is aware of roughly when it's more likely to occur and so prepares himself by putting his hands under his legs, and tensing up. But it's a revelation for him to discover that if he removes these strategies and tries instead to relax, the tic or habit is less intense. Unfortunately, trying to control tics or habits that are uncontrollable is another example of producing conflicting action. Trying to do too much ends up in conflict and produces frustration about action and performance.

So we have traced John's general background tension and body posture, but we need to look at what he is trying to achieve in the situation. What purposeful activity, what project is he undertaking? What is this goal? We can ask what parts of his body he is tensing and how the tension in his arm, chest, and shoulder fits into this preparation. Maybe it doesn't, but it could be that he is recruiting unnecessary muscles due to habit. Or it could be he is tensing the relevant muscles unnecessarily. So we need to step back and see how John is setting himself up to experience tension and distributing tension. Something very important is how John feels about approaching the situation. Is he happy, concerned, and excited? This is important because our emotions are tied up closely with our body movements. There is a coupling between feeling and movements.

At the planning level, we can be preparing action for two distinct and often conflicting goals; for example, to perform a task both as quickly as accurately as possible, or to be as automated and controlled as possible. I could be preparing to carry out a correct action in the wrong way, since what to do and how to do it are separate stages of motor operation. I could prepare the wrong muscles, or prepare more muscles than necessary, or put too much effort into preparation. There could then be problems with feedback guiding actions in the course of movement. The wrong modality of feedback could be used as information, or modalities of feedback could give conflicting information. The movement system could inform the brain that the body position is fine, but the visual system could signal the position needs correction, whilst the feeling system could be saying the feel of the whole task is not correct. It is important to rely on correct sense criteria and movement indices for an accurate performance. Overpreparation may be an attempt to seek feedback from proprioceptive sources—in other words, an attempt to rely too much on the feeling of effort rather than the concrete visuospatial outcome to know if a task is complete.

There could be conflict between feed forward and feedback systems: the feed forward systems forging ahead and preparing for a stage of action not yet reached, whilst the feedback system feeds back information from a previous stage. Then there is conflict between an automated action wishing to advance quickly to the point of no return and the controlled system holding back, saying "not yet." For example, if I carry out a complex action too quickly and forcibly, I may not have the chance to correct the subtle eye–hand coordination, and I will experience more of a "feeling" type of feedback. A small amount of these conflicts is not a big deal since, in any case, it is impossible to activate just one muscle or one mode of action in complete isolation, and there is likely to be some redundancy of movement and interplay of conflicting sources in all our actions. (Table 6.4A indicates the connection between tension, thinking, and emotion. The client should fill in Table 6.4B to establish his or her personal connection.)

But excessive conflict in muscle use and preparation can lead to suboptimal performance. In the worst case, it can paralyze movement or lead to chronic sustained tension. Subjectively speaking, when we do not perform as we intend, we often experience impatience, frustration, or even rage. This emotion of course then further compounds the blocked action, since we are likely to try to force our action and hence make the system more unstable and out of control. Under some circumstances, particularly when too much effort is applied, or there is a conflict of goals and planning, which does not lead naturally to execution, the muscle system then tries to correct itself. This correction most effectively takes the form

Table 6.4A Illustrating the mutual interactions between mind, muscles, and emotion

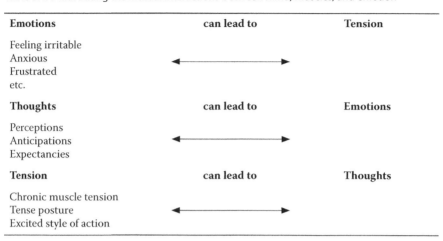

Emotions	can lead to	Tension
Feeling irritable Anxious Frustrated etc.		
Thoughts	**can lead to**	**Emotions**
Perceptions Anticipations Expectancies		
Tension	**can lead to**	**Thoughts**
Chronic muscle tension Tense posture Excited style of action		

Table 6.4B Your personal examples

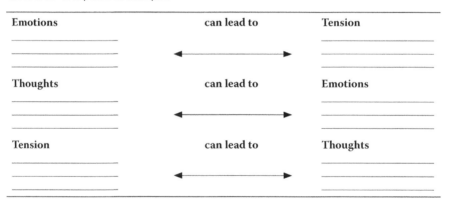

Emotions	can lead to	Tension
Thoughts	**can lead to**	**Emotions**
Tension	**can lead to**	**Thoughts**

of tense–release cycles and these, when overlearned and habitual, can become tics or habits. We have noted already that people with tics or habits tend to over-invest in their movement: often they exert too much effort in a task, or they use irrelevant muscle groups to complete the task or they try to do too much, or try to carry out two tasks at the same time. Such conflict produces chronic tension, which in turn leads to tense–release tic or habit cycles to release the tension (see Figure 6.2, which illustrates flexibility exercises to overcome conflicts).

Take Frank, for example. He is determined not to be late for an appointment, but on the other hand he hates to waste time, so he wants to do as much as possible before leaving for the appointment but does not want to arrive too early. So he uses his time until the last possible minute to leave for the appointment. He ends up rushing to the appointment in automated fashion. But in this automated mode, he is now not well equipped to deal with unforeseen events on the way. He finds it difficult to negotiate a correction in his action plan due to a road closure or an accident. He cannot easily implement a change in attitude, since he has the idea he must arrive on time as quickly as possible. His feedback mode is relying on feel rather than visual environmental cues. So he gets into a frustration–action cycle rather than re-orienting and revising his action. The frustration makes him try even more to adapt circumstances to his plans of rushing to the appointment. So he becomes tenser. As a consequence, his face muscles tighten, perhaps because he feels like cursing or complaining. But these muscles are not useful in his rushing around, so they just stay tense and prepared for action. The tension leaves the face muscles in a stage of constant preparation, and a tense–release cycle ensues, which maintains the preparation and tension.

This quick tense–release cycle becomes the tic or habit, and its role is to recalibrate the muscle tension to permit it to remain tense and prepared. The frustration–action conflict then can be set up by an initial attitude "I must do things this way," "the time cannot be changed," "it's impossible for me to be late," which subsequently confounds the flexibility required for the feedforward intentional stage of planning action.

Another way in which surplus effort can show itself is by the client keeping emotions, sentiments, and assertions in, holding his or her tongue and not expressing them, perhaps for fear of consequences or just because they are considered inappropriate. People with tics and habits are often plagued with both impulses and inhibitions. They feel they should say a word or carry out a deed but then put the brakes on because a voice says don't do it. This holding in inevitably leads to tension and frustration. As an example: I should express myself but I feel I shouldn't. The tension this creates may stay around a lot longer, past the moment of the inhibition.

Unhelpful Attempts at Self-management of Tics or Habits

Acute awareness of potentially negative judgments regarding tics or habits can lead people with tics or habits to attempt to suppress, delay, or disguise their tics or habits, often with a view to hiding them from others. Unfortunately, common strategies useful in resisting tics or habits can also cause conflict and tension. Common strategies include trying to suppress the tic or habit by tensing muscles antagonistic to the tic or habit muscles, tensing the whole area where the tic or habit occurs, modifying one's posture, delaying the tic or habit, and attempting to disguise the tic or habit with other movements (Wojcieszek & Lang, 1995). These strategies commonly result in increased muscular tension and thus a renewed impetus to tic or habit. Often, and this applies particularly to habits, there are attempts to escape or avoid certain emotions because the person cannot deal with them or is trying to fight them. So the client's thoughts and beliefs about how to act may be sabotaging the client's movements (see Table 6.5).

The strategies induce a constant state of overpreparation—like preparing to catch a ball that is never thrown to you. Tension is released naturally by a tense–release cycle, which nonetheless maintains the tension chronically.

Table 6.5 Sample of self-sabotaging tension producing strategies to suppress tics or habits

Wearing heavy or baggy clothes	Willing it not to happen
Resisting and keeping it in	Manually holding in
Holding breath for a bit	Saying and repeating no
Avoidance	Substituting for the tic or habit-affected muscle
Distraction by thought or deed	Inhibiting the movement by suppressing it

Table 6.6 Overcoming everyday conflicts through mindfulness

Everyday conflicts interrupting flow	Mindful approach going with the flow
Trying to do five tasks	Perform less than two tasks at once
Speaking on the phone while wanting to finish housework	Focus on how worry about the future is producing sensation in the present.
Impatient with someone because mind is on the next task	Focus on the origins of tension in the present due to impatience.
Waiting for someone while wanting to get ahead	Consciously calm self-thoughts and release tension and tune into the here and now.

To make things easier we have supplied a list of potential strategies the client may use to suppress the tic or habit in Table 6.6. The client can mark the ones that are relevant. This is important because, as we explained in the model, our aim is to remove negative strategies of control by resistance and suppression, which create tension, and replace them with calm control of processes creating tension.

Mindful Engagement

Mindful engagement goes along with flow. To be mindful, the person is fully engaged in their task, connected to the here and now, and aware of surroundings in the here and now. He or she is able to filter stray thoughts and distractions arising from inner mental life. In performing an action mindfully the person is aware of using appropriate tensions focused on a single goal and moving ahead with flow in the action. There is no conflict or inhibition and the action is smooth. This flow can be achieved by bringing mind and body together and performing an act with one goal, one intention, and using the right muscles. It sometimes helps to slow down an action to make it less abrupt. Flow is effecting the directed action simply and smoothly with one aim in view.

When the client performs an action, does he or she always have a clear intention to act and a well-defined goal, or, is he or she frequently distracted en route becoming unfocused? Is the client present in the here and now rather than off in the past or the future in his or her mind? Is the client flexible enough to be able to countermand an action and change course depending on feedback? Is the client using the right amount of effort and the right muscle groups or is he or she tensing unnecessarily?

Anticipations and expectations are always in the future. So we use our imagination to predict what we believe is most likely to occur. The problem is that our expectations may be strongly biased by what happened in a long distant episode in the past that has no connection with current reality. But this expectation will cloud our judgment and make us prepare for the action inefficiently.

Mindfulness Exercises

There are seven attitudinal factors.

Non-judgmental

We are constantly judging and commenting on our own experience and interpreting it as good or bad. It is important to recognize this judging quality of mind and assume the stance of impartial witness and just observe. Take a flexible stance and don't overcomplicate.

Patience

Practicing patience reminds us that we don't have to fill up our time with activity or thinking in order to function. In fact, just the opposite is true, and we need to be more open and let things unfold in their own time to profit to the full.

Receptive mind

Being receptive to new possibilities prevents us becoming stuck in rigidity and the rut of our own assumptions and predictions about life.

Trust

Trust in our own senses means we don't need to put in any extra effort to seeing or hearing. We can confidently take responsibility for ourselves and our decisions and learn to trust our own judgments. Trusting yourself and others is less effort than distrusting.

Non-striving

Non-striving involves simply paying attention to what is happening around you and in your own body without fighting it or resisting it, or just accepting where you are and being in the here and now, rather than striving toward another state.

Along with non-striving goes *acceptance*, which does not mean you have to like everything or accept things the way they are. This attitude sets the stage for acting on a clearer picture of the actual state of affairs. Instead of trying, for example, desperately to go to sleep and sabotaging the process of naturally sleeping, there is a process of letting go. This means letting go of unnecessary effort and investing less in grasping and pushing away. Letting go means not maintaining tension and preparation past its sell by date and also not hanging on to critical, judgmental thoughts as though they are eternal permanent truths that transcend context; likewise, unfulfilled desires that stay around to haunt us and just cause frustration and self-dissatisfaction.

Mindfulness practice; mindful breathing

- Breathing.
- Sit comfortably.
- Eyes closed.
- Focus on your respiration.
- Place your hand on your abdomen and feel the hand move up and down as you breathe.
- Follow your breath as it goes in and out.
- Do not try to force it; let the air go in and out naturally.
- Continue for 15 min.
- Become conscious only of your breath.
- Your mind will wander; if it does simply observe it and accept that is what minds do.
- Bring the mind back to the breath.

Breathing is a basic function and focusing on breathing lets us focus on a natural life function and natural rhythm like the sea. It can be mesmerizing and excludes other noises.

You can master this focus on sensations in different parts of your body at the same time as continuing to breathe in and out with your natural rhythm.

Imagine your consciousness is in your breath and you are directing your attention by directing your breath to different parts of your body.

Mindful sensory focus

Examine the different sensations in your hands, the back of your feet, in particular spots of your body you are not usually aware of. Imagine your consciousness is a microscope zooming in on all the noises of the body no matter how small or distant the location. Be aware of the quality of the sensations, let your conscious relate to and get to know the feel of each body part, and with your breath try to give new life to each part with your out breath.

You can apply these exercises to daily living be it: eating, walking, dealing with a problem, or cleaning your teeth. The same mindful strategies apply:

- Focusing on the minutiae of the activity as it occurs in the here and now.
- Focusing on your reactions and feelings, observing the actions and movements, creating a distance, and focusing on the resources you are using in the action. If your mind wanders, accept the wandering and wonder at the natural flow of the action adopting a compassionate and kind mind to the actions you are focused on.

After covering the content of this chapter the client should understand the importance of muscle flexibility and the causes of muscle conflict, and now we move on to other exercises to improve flexibility.

Therapist checklist for tension before ticking

The client understands the origins of tension in muscle use and the link with the brain	Yes / No ❏ ❏
The client understands the ways tensions arise through muscle use and the importance of muscle flexibility, and knows how redundant muscle tension does not go away	Yes / No ❏ ❏
The client can identify conflicts in everyday life in the way action is prepared	Yes / No ❏ ❏
The client knows how unhelpful attempts to suppress tics encourage them	Yes / No ❏ ❏
The client is aware of how preparing informs performance, how inhibition impairs performance, and flow comes from not inhibiting, but smooth planning	Yes / No ❏ ❏
The client experiences how mindfulness and flow improve engagement and optimal performance	Yes / No ❏ ❏

7

Increasing Flexibility

In this chapter we continue with exploring movement flexibility and physical flexibility, more systematically. First, in the tic- or habit-affected muscle to improve use, and to attain greater muscle control over the tic or habit; second, over all the body; and finally, over our reactions to sensations. Our tension depends also on our thinking and approach to situations, and our beliefs and assumptions underpin the way we undertake activities.

Discriminating Muscle Contractions

We have talked a lot about preventing the buildup of tension and dealing with unnecessary activation, and mentioned that there is both a cognitive and physiological part to this buildup. Here we deal systematically with the physiological part (muscles and sensations). The exercises are in continuity with the last chapter, where we have already covered learning to use the correct muscles for the correct job—in other words not activating redundant muscles. Correct muscle use requires monitoring activity during a task and perhaps slowing it down and checking for where redundant muscles are activated due to habit or misuse.

The second exercise aims to increase the flexibility of the muscles so that they don't jump into tense mode so easily, and we do this by becoming aware of and modifying the tension buildup in each muscle using exercises we call discrimination exercises. What we mean by discrimination is that people learn to contract their muscles, particularly tic- or habit-affected muscles, gradually across the range of tension so they do not jump from 0–100% tension. We have found in our research that tic-affected muscles tend to be more brittle and jumpy. There are various ways of completing the discrimination exercises including use of biofeedback apparatus to give objective feedback on gauging tension by use of the hand or a mirror. It is important to link the flexibility of each range with a sensation that allows the person to identify when the muscle is 50% or so contracted, but, in particular, when it is becoming tense and before it has jumped to 100%. It is not necessary to identify every degree of tension, just to develop awareness of when it is 25%, 50%, or 75% contracted.

Managing Tic and Habit Disorders: A Cognitive Psychophysiological Approach with Acceptance Strategies, First Edition. Kieron P O'Connor, Marc E Lavoie, and Benjamin Schoendorff.
© 2017 John Wiley & Sons, Ltd. Published 2017 by John Wiley & Sons, Ltd.
Companion Website: www.wiley.com/go/oconnor/managingticandhabitdsorders

The first part of becoming more flexible in the use of muscle contraction is to learn to discriminate muscle use and to localize actions to the correct muscle groups and not involve redundant muscles (see Chapter 6). One problem we have noted previously is that tension can often be produced by activating non-relevant muscles; for example, tensing the face when lifting a glass. This redundant tension may be because clients are preparing for more than one action or may just be a tension developed through habit. The problem is that because this tension is not useful it does not adapt but hangs around as tension. The client could practice with the therapist and at home in performing certain actions including actions linked with a high risk of ticking to see if the client recruits redundant muscles. We gave a list of efficient actions and muscle use in Table 6.1. We noted in Chapter 6 how John tenses his body, with tension in his arm, chest, and shoulder. It could be that he is recruiting unnecessary muscles due to habit. Or it could be he is tensing the relevant muscles unnecessarily. Or his muscles are simply not flexible enough to relax, which brings us to the discrimination. Luckily there are exercises to help muscles become more flexible.

Here we have systemized these exercises to directly influence muscle activity and we start with the principal muscle or muscle groups identified with the principal tic or habit. By now the client should have identified the muscle principally involved in the problem and any other muscles considered to be involved. The discrimination exercises train the client to better discriminate and recognize the state of tension–relaxation in the muscle. Doing the exercises inevitably changes the nature of the muscle movement and sometimes affects the intensity of the tic or habit.

In order to *discriminate* between different muscle states the client is encouraged to learn to *isolate* the muscle, and then contract and relax it *slowly*, moving from a state of tension to one of relaxation, passing gradually through the different stages of tension. In doing this slowly the client will gain more flexibility in control of the muscle and will be able to identify different states of contraction of the muscle. The muscle itself will also become more flexible. We have found that muscles involved in tics and habits tend to be more rigid and less flexible than other muscles and so their owners have more problems tensing them slowly and regularly. Most people with tics and habits are more affected on one side of the body than the other. We suggest the client practice the discrimination exercises on both sides. The client will find the less affected side easier to control. If both sides are equally affected the client should choose a non-affected muscle and practice the exercises on this side as a reference guide to compare with the affected muscle. Indeed, we suggest the exercises are practiced first in the non-tic-affected muscles (maybe the symmetrically opposite muscle) because the existing flexibility will be greater and therefore the will be exercises easier and will form a point of comparison to the tic- or habit-affected muscles.

Rationale and Procedure for Discrimination Exercises

Muscles are under our voluntary control and we can thus decide to voluntarily contract or relax a muscle. By relaxing the tension in the muscles, we give the signal to our whole body to relax; we can replace the symptoms of anxiety and tension with calm and relief. However, before learning how to relax muscular tension, it is initially necessary to learn how to recognize it. The discrimination exercises hence represent a significant element in the client's relaxation training. It is by practicing these exercises that the client will be able to detect the difference between the presence and the absence of tension and to detect the various levels of contraction.

The aim of the discrimination and relaxation exercises is to solidify control and awareness of muscle tension so that the client becomes more aware of when tic- or habit-affected muscles are tensing. The discrimination exercises apply to the principal tic-affected muscle (the most implicated muscle, which contracts first) and opposite muscles that are not affected (symmetrical) and act as a reference point.

The procedure to follow in discrimination is first to contract and relax the muscle as slowly as possible. So, if the client has an eye tic he or she should try opening and closing the eyes as gently and slowly as possible. If the client has a shoulder twitch, he or she should raise and lower the shoulder slowly. If the client has a habit, he or she should relax and contract the hand involved slowly. To begin with, the client may focus on three levels: no tension; half-tension (50%); and full tension. After the client has mastered this, he or she should try to isolate the contraction as much as possible so that only the muscle directly relevant is being moved. Also, check that no other unnecessary muscles near or far are involved other than those that are necessary. The client can check tension by feel or use of hands for feedback, or by identifying the sensations through mental associations. By contracting and relaxing slowly, the ability to detect the tension eventually at five different levels (0, 25%, 50%, 75%, and 100%) will develop naturally. Under no circumstances force the muscle contraction, rather tense it gently.

Each week, for the next 2 weeks, the client is encouraged to practice the discrimination exercises. In order to do the exercises, the client should install him or herself comfortably in an armchair and follow the instructions. Each exercise will be repeated twice. The muscle contraction should be maintained for 5 s and the relaxation gradually carried over a 10-s period. The client should remember, as much as possible, to associate breath expiration with muscular relaxation. Moreover, as the client decontracts the muscle, try to encourage awareness of the various feelings connected to the three and eventually five levels of tension, and in particular encourage the client to notice the difference between tensing and decontracting. It is generally easier to tense the muscle from 0–25–50–75–100% than to relax it through the same levels.

Note: The discrimination exercises are not relaxation exercises, in that the aim is to increase flexibility, gain knowledge of tension, improve control, and instruct on the proper use of the muscles with appropriate contractions for the job in hand.

We ask clients to try to identify when the muscle is completely tense, half-tense, and then fully tense (roughly). When the client has mastered this gradient of tensing ask him or her to try to find the midpoint between relaxed and half-relaxed, and between half-relaxed and fully tense. At odd times throughout the day ask the client to check and see if he or she can identify what level of tension is present in this muscle: relaxed, half-relaxed, or tense. Repeat the discrimination exercise with the client to check whether the client was correct

Table 7.1 Discrimination exercise

Muscle: _____	Flexibility (0–50–100): _____
Date: _____	Flexibility (0–25–50–75–100): _____
Muscle: _____	Flexibility (0–50–100): _____
Date: _____	Flexibility (0–25–50–75–100): _____
Muscle: _____	Flexibility (0–50–100): _____
Date: _____	Flexibility (0–25–50–75–100): _____
Muscle: _____	Flexibility (0–50–100): _____
Date: _____	Flexibility (0–25–50–75–100): _____
Muscle: _____	Flexibility (0–50–100): _____
Date: _____	Flexibility (0–25–50–75–100): _____
Muscle: _____	Flexibility (0–50–100): _____
Date: _____	Flexibility (0–25–50–75–100): _____
Muscle: _____	Flexibility (0–50–100): _____
Date: _____	Flexibility (0–25–50–75–100): _____

in the detection. We provide a form to fill in to monitor the discrimination exercise progress on a daily basis (see Table 7.1).

Discrimination with habits

Mostly the muscle implicated will be in the hand or arm. So the exercises can be performed here, check from your observation which muscle tenses the most and soonest, and choose appropriately.

Discrimination with complex tics

Choose the muscle that tenses soonest and first at the beginning of the sequence.

Phonic tics

Slow down the sound and try to modulate the intensity of the volume according to the range of levels. Also, apply the exercises to the diaphragm and muscles controlling the breathing and the level of tension in face muscles at the same time.

Mental tics

Slow down the sequence of the counting or jumping; notice what muscles you are tensing abruptly or intensely at the same time (jaw, eyes, face, legs).Usually there are movements associated with mental tics. Control the sequence and intensity or rapidity, depending on what is most appropriate, and do this mentally until you can control the speed of the mental tic.

The discrimination exercise should be repeated until: (a) the client can accurately detect the level of tension (0–25–50–75–100%) in the tic- or habit-affected muscle; (b) the client can contract and relax the muscle slowly, smoothly, and individually; and (c) the client is more conscious of the muscle contraction and tension onset before the tic or habit or movement arises (Table 7.1 provides a practice sheet for the discrimination exercise).

Whole Body Muscle Control

The next stage is tension control and relaxation of the whole body. Discrimination is not relaxation but the discrimination helps establish flexibility for relaxation training. Relaxation takes time and is a learning process usually divided into four stages.

The exercises aim to make the client aware of tension buildup in his or her body and where principal tensions arise, and then release them. After practicing these exercises the client will be able to scan his or her body and prevent buildup of tension. Slowly the client will learn to act more calmly and flexibly with the whole body and avoid conflict in preparation; he or she will be able to detect tension anywhere and let it go.

Muscle Relaxation

Actually the body can never be in an absolute state of relaxation, and what's more, many other muscle states beside relaxation, such as stretching or warming, can have an effect on tension. Relaxation is also about feeling comfortable with the posture and with the way different muscles are coordinating with each other, and how the action is flowing. It is not always possible or necessary to relax each muscle absolutely, so we recommend an applied relaxation training that involves using muscles in a relaxed but active way in a variety of everyday postures and situations, whilst nonetheless following principles of slow graded contraction and relaxation muscle action.

The method involves:

1) Learning to breathe better and mastering breath control.
2) Learning to isolate tension and to let go in different muscles.
3) Learning to detect tension as soon as possible to prevent its buildup.
4) Applying the relaxation even when active and in motion.

We begin the relaxation exercises with attention to breathing. Table 7.2 provides an exercise sheet for the relaxation exercises.

Table 7.2 Diary record of relaxation

Date Time	Feel tension (where)	Performed relaxation exercises

Date Time	Feel tension (where)	Performed relaxation exercises

Check the Breathing, Posture, and Flow During Movement

Now examine client breathing when moving. People often stop breathing when they move, or start breathing in an irregular fashion. We deal with this later more generally under relaxation. But make a note of situations where the client notices any change in his or her breathing. How does the client breathe during the onset of the problem? Breathing patterns should have been recognized when observing the tic or habit.

Breathe Better

When they get tense many people find that they also stop breathing or breathe in an irregular fashion. Has the client noticed how he or she breathes when the habit or tic occurs? An essential part of relaxation is breathing fully and freely.

There are two elements to consider: (a) the ratio of in breath to out breath; and (b) which muscles the client uses in breathing.

The aim of breathing is to take in oxygen, which is converted into energy. A functioning system takes in what it needs and expels what it does not need. Optimally the lungs should be full after inspiration to allow efficient absorption. When we are stressed, we often breathe shallowly because everything around the throat, neck, and shoulders is constricted. Just by filling the lungs the client can ease some of this tension, and anyway establishing a normal flow of air relaxes the client. When the client breathes in, he or she should feel that the ribcage expands, particularly that the upper back expands since this is where the lungs are located.

Then he or she should breathe in to the count of 1, 2, 3, pause.

Breathe out to the count of 1, 2, 3, 4, pause.

Ask the client to make a noise on the out breath to give feedback on the slow count on the out breath. Repeat this deep slow breathing twice a day for six times each and before doing the full relaxation exercises.

The client might feel dizzy at first—stop if necessary. With gradual practice of the exercises, the dizziness should clear, but if it continues this may mean the client is breathing too quickly or inhaling more air than he or she is exhaling. If the client has a vertigo problem, he or she may wish to seek medical advice on the exercises. Whenever the client finds him or herself breathing irregularly, he or she should repeat the exercise to improve the breathing and bring a sense of calm in stressful situations.

An exercise that may help breathing is *laughter yoga*. In this the person takes an in and out breath using the abdomen, laughing on the out breath. The laughter on the out breath is feedback through the expulsion of air and noise. Laughter also increases well-being and even forced laughter can aid stress reduction (Kataria, 2012).

Relaxation Exercises

The aim of the relaxation exercises is for the client to become more and more conscious of when the tension begins to build up so that he or she can prevent it before it starts. The key phrase here is: *the tension is never at the point the client first detects it*, the tension usually builds up before awareness, and one of the goals here is early detection. After following the exercises the client will begin to detect the tension coming earlier and earlier and realize that what he or she thought was the onset of the tension was in fact the mid-point in the buildup of the tension.

When practicing the exercises, it is important to be attentive to the following points:

1) Make sure the client is tensing the muscle in the correct way and does not *over*tense it, or he or she may get aches or cramps.
2) Ensure the client is in a comfortable position free from distraction and that he or she is able to direct thoughts entirely to the exercises.

3) Check that the client is breathing correctly during the exercises.
4) Practice the exercises for the times given; do not overpractice, particularly when the client is just beginning.

In the next section we list the principal muscles and how to tense and relax them. The initial tension–relaxation exercises in all muscles involve four cycles.

Cycle 1

1) Breathe in.
2) Tense muscle, slowly counting to five.
3) Keep tense for a further 5 s.
4) Relax muscle slowly over 5 s.
5) Breathe out at the same time.

The exercise in this cycle is similar to the discrimination exercise and it is important for the client to recognize the difference between tension and relaxation. Repeat Cycle 1 six times so the client will become familiar with it and also feel more relaxed.

Cycle 2

1) Tense the muscle again but now check how many other muscles are also tense, either near or far from the muscle you are tensing.
2) Repeat the tense–relax exercise as in Cycle 1 but isolate the activity as far as possible to the one muscle involved.

Repeat these two cycles for each muscle listed below in the upper and lower body, twice a day.

Forearm (right and left individually)
Cycle 1:
  Tense: Clench fists with thumb outside. Breathe in: 1, 2, 3, 4, 5.
  Relax: Unfold fists till fingers are loose. Breathe out: 1, 2, 3, 4, 5.
Cycle 2:
  Check redundant tension in: biceps, shoulders, jaw, and legs.
  Let go and isolate fists.

Upper arm (right and left individually)
Cycle 1:
  Tense: Bring forearm up to shoulder and press upper arm close to your body.
  Relax: Let forearm hang loose.
Cycle 2:
  Check for other unnecessary tensions in: cheek, mouth, chin, neck, and shoulders.
  Isolate the forearm.

Shoulders I

Cycle 1:

>Tense: Raise both shoulders toward the ears trying to get them as high as possible.

>Relax: Let them drop again and hang a little forward.

Cycle 2:

>Check for other unnecessary tensions in: jaw, mouth, and abdomen.

>Isolate shoulders.

Shoulders II

Cycle 1:

>Tense: As in shoulder I, but as you lift rotate the shoulders a little to the back.

>Relax: As you relax rotate them to the front.

Neck I

Cycle 1:

>Tense: Press chin down until back of neck is stretched; push chin back so that head moves backwards.

>Relax: Lift chin up so that head goes back and down and head is hanging back on the shoulders.

Cycle 2:

>Check for other unnecessary tensions: e.g., face.

>Isolate neck.

Neck II

>Repeat Neck I but lean head left to one side at an angle, and then repeat with head leant right at an angle.

Jaw

Cycle 1:

>Tense: Push jaw up to mouth creating tension in muscles next to the ears.

>Relax: Open mouth, let jaw drop, and waggle it about left–right, back and forth.

Cycle 2:

>Check for other unnecessary tensions: e.g., rest of the face and neck.

>Isolate jaw.

Mouth

Cycle 1:

>Tense: Purse lips together and force tongue against the roof of the mouth.

>Relax: Smile and let the tongue drop to the floor of the mouth.

Cycle 2:

>Check for other unnecessary tensions: e.g., jaw and eyes.

>Isolate lips.

Cheeks (right and left)

Tense: Raise cheek and corner of the mouth toward the eye.

Relax: Bring cheek back to mouth.

Eyes

Tense: Close eyes, bring cheek toward eyebrows.

Relax: Open eyes wide.

Check for other unnecessary tensions.

Isolate eyes.

Forehead

Tense: Frown and wrinkle forehead, bringing eyebrows together.

Relax: Show an expression of surprise and raise eyebrows.

Lower leg (right and left)

Tense: Place feet on the floor and try to push feet together (but without moving feet).

Relax: Feel feet resting on the floor with no effort.

Upper leg (right and left)

Tense: Keep feet on the floor and try to lift knees up (but without moving them).

Relax: Keep legs still and planted on the floor making no conscious effort.

Buttocks

Tense: Try to press the two buttocks together.

Relax: Lean back in the armchair so there is no weight on your buttocks and they are loose.

Abdomen

Tense: Pull abdomen in and up until you feel a "knot" there.

Relax: Let the abdomen expand out as though it has a balloon in it.

Posture

Tense: Stand up feet apart, tense all limb muscles at the same time.

Relax: Then untense the limbs, and imagine a string through your center pulling you up. You should ideally be balanced around your center of gravity—nothing sticking out forwards or backwards.

Cycle 3

The client should practice all these relaxation exercises in total twice a day (at end and start) for 1 week until they have become familiar. Then he or she should speed up the tense–relax cycle to just 1–2 s in total for each muscle for the next week. Finally, at the end of the week, instead of doing the exercises, the client should check that each muscle is relaxed and just repeat a word like "relax" to him or herself to ensure that each muscle is in its proper relaxed state.

If there is a particular scene or image that the client associates with relaxation, you may use that to help him or her relax instead of using a word.

Cycle 4

The final stage is for the client to move from relaxing when the muscles are static to relaxing when they are dynamic and the body is in everyday motion. The client should practice using the ability he or she has developed to check his or her own muscles and detect tension and relax, whilst performing the actions given in Table 6.2. It's more difficult when the client is moving about or doing a task to focus on what state his or her body is in, but it's just a case of dividing attention as we discussed earlier. Eventually, the client will find checking that he or she is relaxed will become automatic.

Refocusing Sensations

In this exercise, we combine the skills the client has acquired in relaxation and awareness to address other aspects of unnecessary activation and stimulation. Although our sensations and moving are separate events, often they are tied together so that when we feel bad or irritated, this affects the way we move around.

In the case of sensations, the same connection applies. Many people with tics or habits describe a hypersensibility to sensation or touch, or experience uncomfortable tingling or warm rushes in their limbs and elsewhere. For example, Joan would frequently experience tingling sensations up and down her legs, which made it difficult for her to sit still. Other clients report suddenly being aware of focus spots or tensions that appear prior to or at the same time as tics. These can occur sometime before tic or habit onset, or they can occur immediately preceding tic or habit onset. Many interpret this as an urge to tic or habit. In either case, after experiencing the urge, the person is likely to feel that the tic or habit is inevitable and react accordingly. But if we look at the reaction, we see that in many ways the reaction to the urge makes the urge a self-fulfilling prophesy. People tense up, or try to suppress the sensation, or act and prepare as though the tic or habit onset is inevitable.

Similarly, when experiencing a tingling sensation, Joan has a tendency to move around, fidget, or change position to try to contain the movement. Recall what we said earlier about viewing behaviors that maintain the tension level, as false friends. These reactions to sensations fit into this category and maintain higher chronic levels of activation, so the client is likely to experience a vicious circle. The more the client feels obliged to act, react, tense, and move to alleviate these sensations, the more he or she will feel the need to move even more, since movement actually reinforces the need for stimulation. However, if the client just stays calm and relaxed when the sensations arise, the sensation is more likely to decrease and he or she will feel less need for further movement and stimulation—a bit like scratching an itch.

This section covers exercises known as "acceptance exercises" to help the client tolerate better these sensations or premonitory urges. If the client does not react adversely to the sensations, the sensations will go away of their own accord. If the client feels it is useful to pay attention to the sensations, be vigilant, and try to put effort into reacting to them, in order to diminish the impact of the sensations, this will make the sensations more significant and more annoying and the client becomes tenser. So the way to diminish the irritation and importance of the sensations is initially to accept the sensations and not fight or suppress them; validate them as real sensations but not interpret them further. The client can accomplish this result by tolerating the sensation and by not: (a) reacting behaviorally to it; (b) tensing physically; (c) not dwelling on it mentally; and (d) in particular not saying or thinking: "Oh no, here it comes again, I wish it would go away, I'm never going to feel better, this is a terrible feeling, I'm not normal, and so on." Such thinking will exacerbate the problem since the client is giving the sensation a great menacing power that it doesn't really possess unless the client provides it.

It is also important to realize that the power that the client attributes to the sensation is associated with a thinking habit, and so the thought is likely to pop up automatically even before the client is aware of it. For example, a client may find him or herself consciously monitoring a sensation by being vigilant to it, way before the sensation appears. In effect, the best way for the client to ignore the sensation is to do absolutely nothing special when it arises; just carrying on with his or her routine and not react even a little to the onset of the sensation. The client must be careful not to let slip any old habits, such as making even a small change in limb position to accommodate the sensation. In particular, distracting attention from the sensation by focusing on routine will make sure the person is not inadvertently stoking the sensation with thoughts like "Has it gone away yet?" "Is it still here?," which means the client is still giving it special attention. The client can keep a record on the forms below of his or her attempts to modify the intensity of the sensation or premonitory urge by changing reactions, thoughts, and behavior.

If the client finds it difficult to let the sensations go by, distraction or refocusing on another activity may be helpful, but the client should not fight the sensation. They should *not* try to understand it to suppress it, or concentrate on making it disappear, or accept it as a sign.

Description of sensation/urge

Old reactions: When my sensation arises, I have the habit of:
    Behavior: _____
    Emotional reaction: _____
    Attentional reaction: _____
    Thinking about it: _____
    Today I will systematically accept the sensation until it decreases and go about my daily routine and eliminate my usual reactions to the sensation.
    Degree of success in eliminating reactions (0—not successful; 100—very successful): _____

Length of time accepted: _____

Comments: _____

Preventing the problem

The client will now have enough strategies to prevent the buildup of chronic tension and associated sensations at source. Prevention can be effective if clients:

1) Remain aware of his or her state of tension.
2) Practice both the mental and physical exercises to relax his or her state of activation.
3) Persist in regular practice of acceptance of sensations for the next few weeks.

Once the client has practiced sufficiently preventing tension buildup through reactions to sensations, the prevention will become automatic and he or she won't have to exert conscious effort.

Once the client has mastered this acceptance approach he or she can practice mentally relaxing and getting in the right state of mind to relax, and giving him or herself permission to be relaxed, in particular making sure he or she is fully engaged with the exercises and not thinking of something else. As we have noted, thinking can exert an influence on tension and how we relax. So it is important to address thinking flexibility as well as muscle flexibility to ensure that thoughts and beliefs allow the person to relax.

We have already discussed flow of action in Chapter 6. This flow can be achieved by bringing mind and body together and performing an act with one goal, one intention, and the right muscles continually. It sometimes helps to slow down an action to make it less abrupt. Flow is effecting an action simply and smoothly with one aim in view.

Therapist checklist for discrimination and relaxation

The client understands the aim of improving flexibility through the discrimination exercises	Yes / No ❏ ❏
The client practices the exercises regularly on the non-affected side and the affected side	Yes / No ❏ ❏
Meets the criteria of flexibility in affected muscles.	Yes / No ❏ ❏
Practices relaxation: Breathing; progressive relaxation (steps, 1, 2, 3, 4)	Yes / No ❏ ❏
Practices exercises every day and detects preliminary tension	Yes / No ❏ ❏
Practices refocusing sensations exercises and fills in feedback forms	Yes / No ❏ ❏

8

Addressing Styles of Planning Action

In this chapter we deal in more detail with the importance of styles of action, the different ways we prepare for action, and the impact of these styles on tension and emotion and how they are linked to thoughts. We illustrate how styles of preparing for action play a role in tension buildup and tic or habit onset, and how the thoughts inspiring them are often perfectionist not impulsive thoughts. In this chapter we'll review how these different elements can interact, and how thoughts, actions, and emotions feed off one another and can create a cycle of tension that is difficult to break. We'll review different approaches to regulating tension and emotions that will lay the ground work to effective tic and habit control and outline the processes on which to intervene to maximize the chances of breaking the tic or habit cycle.

Style of Planning: Pulling Together Sensory, Emotional, and Motor Aspects of Ticking

Tics or habits often result from excess muscular tension and serve to provide short-term relief from that tension. For all animals, premotor activation or preparation for action is a highly adaptive process that allows fast and appropriate responses to changes in the environment. Premotor activation is key to avoiding predators and catching prey. In humans, due to our highly evolved cognitive abilities, premotor activation can be triggered not only by changes in the physical environment, but also by conscious planning, thoughts, emotions, or memories that at times can seem to appear randomly. For most animals, responding to the appearance of a predator or a prey by increased premotor activation is a transitory response that dies down soon after environmental conditions change again. For humans, however, the inner environment does not change quite so readily. Thoughts and emotions related to danger or strived-for goals can linger well beyond the disappearance of either predator or prey and prevent premotor activation from returning to a resting base rate, causing chronic levels of tension that provide the ideal breeding grounds for tic and habit disorders. Pervasive beliefs about situations, places, or what needs to be done may also play a role as well as the mood, state, and anticipations particular to each situation.

Managing Tic and Habit Disorders: A Cognitive Psychophysiological Approach with Acceptance Strategies, First Edition. Kieron P O'Connor, Marc E Lavoie, and Benjamin Schoendorff.
© 2017 John Wiley & Sons, Ltd. Published 2017 by John Wiley & Sons, Ltd.
Companion Website: www.wiley.com/go/oconnor/managingticandhabitdsorders

When an action is anticipated and planned, we imagine what effort and type of action may be required. Some of this process may have become automatic with practice, for example, when it comes to common actions such as walking up a flight of stairs, and as for when we plan to lift a box we have been told is heavy. Before we grab the box and lift, we will tense muscles at a level appropriate to the effort required by the task. Imagine now that, contrary to what the client was told, the box is in fact empty and very light. The client will naturally readjust the tension in his or her arm muscles as his or her brain receives feedback that the task does not require much tension to be completed.

This sensory–motor feedback loop operates in part outside of conscious awareness but can be impacted by conscious action. In the lighter-than-imagined box example, the difference between expected required muscle tone and actually required muscle tone is so large that the adjustment itself is perceptible. In most everyday actions, however, this feedback is automatic. People with tic and habit disorders may be subject to a failing in this feedback loop, both conscious and unconscious. As a result, muscle tension is less often down-regulated when not required, and people with a tic or habit become unable to perceive residual levels of muscular tension, leading to chronic tension and the need to relieve it through tics or the disordered habit.

In some senses, people with tics or habits approach every task as if it were a hard-to-lift super-heavy box that has to be moved as fast as possible. They will overplan their actions, imagine them as being more complicated than they are, and expend too much energy doing them. Thoughts and emotions may be implicated in elevated levels of muscular tension. Thoughts, emotions, and muscle activation all have an impact on one another.

Styles of Action

In our research, we have identified three main styles of planning and of action involved in tic and habit disorders: overcomplication, overpreparation, and overactivity.

Each style of action involves behavioral and cognitive facets. Many of the behavioral aspects of the client's styles of action are reflected in responses to the completed STOP questionnaire, which can often be the starting point for identifying everyday styles. Using the STOP questionnaire will help the client's identify their personalized styles of planning and action (Table 8.1). Three main factors have emerged from the scale, *overpreparing*, *overcomplicating*, and *overactivity*. The first factor is planning to do too much, the second if adding in unnecessary detail or movements, and the third is trying to squeeze as much as possible into the time available. Clients may show more than one style, and it is common to find overpreparation going hand in hand with overcomplication.

Overcomplicating can make even simple tasks seem complicated and clients imagine unforeseen eventualities and are prone to getting side-tracked as they carry out a task. Therefore, a task may take longer due to the tendency to add in

Table 8.1 Style of action

Personalized style of action

unnecessary components or adopting a roundabout way of completing the task. Overcomplicating also involves a tendency to go into unnecessary detail that could make the task seem more complex, or accomplishing a task and thinking of how it can be embellished by doing extra, or getting side-tracked, or analyzing the task for hidden elements.

Overpreparing clients will try and plan the action down to the slightest detail and they will approach it with heightened levels of tension, as if every task were a super-heavy box to lift. Overpreparation *always* involves using more effort than is necessary, whether emotional, physical, or intellectual effort. Overpreparation also involves using surplus and/or redundant muscles and effort, getting too emotionally involved, or the opposite—putting a lot of effort into suppressing and keeping emotions in rather than expressing them normally. It may imply effort put into playing a role rather than acting naturally, or overattending and overstraining the body to hear or see someone. Overpreparing could also mean relying on muscular cues or bodily feelings of fatigue or effort to know if a task has been accomplished.

Overactive clients will tend to do many tasks at once, overload themselves with tasks, and try to accomplish more in a task than is necessary to perform well. When doing a task, they may always be thinking of the next steps ahead rather than focusing on the task at hand. They might find it difficult to stay still and have nothing to do. They might feel impatient having to queue for services. They will worry about what people think of them, how they are seen and judged, adding to the level of tension going into an action. They might appear to be always in a hurry and their speech might be compressed or hurried. Overactivity often involves: trying to accomplish too much, taking on too much, and always making sure one is too occupied, often fruitlessly. It also involves always being ahead of oneself and so never focusing fully on the task in hand because attention is always distracted by anticipation of the next task; plus a physical ability to talk too fast and move too quickly and an inability to keep still for long.

Once the clients personal style(s) has been identified in Table 8.1, and verified according to the STOP categories in Table 8.2, invite them to carry out a cost–benefit analysis of their style(s) of action in Table 8.3.

Table 8.2 Personal styles of action

Personal style of action	Category	Description	Overpreparation, etc.

Table 8.3 Behavioral benefit and cost calculation for personal styles of action

Personalized style of action	Benefit	Cost

1 point for every cost: _____

1 point for every benefit: _____

Total costs: _____

Total benefits: _____

Ratio of benefits to costs: benefit/costs = _____

Behavioral Cost

There is a behavioral cost to adopting these styles of action. They do not achieve the effect desired. Generally they prevent the client from being present in the here and now, they cause undue tensions and stress, they disallow the client to perform at best capacity, are usually tiresome, and generate a feeling of lack of success by for example attempting too much and failing. We can calculate with the client the costs and benefits of each personalized style of action and assess the efficiency of these styles of action and whether they are adaptive or maladaptive according to their behavioral cost. In doing so the therapist considers any of the client's personal styles of action (overcomplicating, overpreparing, overactivity) through questioning the client and by reference to the STOP questionnaire, and calculates with the client what is termed the cost effectiveness of the style in order to calculate the behavioral costs. Cost effectiveness analysis involves listing apparent advantages of the style of action alongside the costs and disadvantages, and behavioral cost can be calculated in Table 8.3.

The client will find that many of his or her maladaptive strategies have one of the following negative side effects: an overactive style of action in which the person tries to do too much at once and expends too much effort might impair regulation of arousal and attention. This leads to, and is reinforced by, restlessness. These deficits in regulating arousal and attention lead many tic or habit sufferers to experience difficulties in initiating and carrying through complex tasks requiring controlled allocation of resources. This can lead to frustration both in anticipation and in relation to the consequences of complex task performance, particularly for tasks requiring open loop planning (i.e., controlled rather than automated regulation). The associated emotions at the time of onset of tics or habits are frustration, impatience, and dissatisfaction. High levels of felt frustration might contribute to distracting people with tic and habit disorders from the visuo-spatial cues that could best serve to regulate action and movement planning, and lead them to rely more on interoceptive cues, that is, what they are feeling rather than what they can perceive with their five senses.

Overpreparation could render the person less able to identify when enough genuine effort has been invested or when an action has been completed. In turn, frustration and impatience feed tension and create another loop of tense–release–retense. In this way muscles are continually overreadied for action in an action–frustration cycle that keeps them in a chronic state of overpreparation. Overcomplication may lead the person off into irrelevant details and impede or even paralyze performance.

Overactive persons will always be in a rush, have trouble relaxing, and feel in the grip of conflicts about what activity to devote time and energy to at any given moment. They will habitually feel stressed, irritable, and rarely satisfied with what they do, which will negatively impact their sense of self. As noted, the overpreparation dimension of the scale denotes investing too much physical, intellectual, or emotional energy into any given task. On a physical level, this will often take the form of recruiting unnecessary muscle groups to perform an action. For example, an action such as lifting a pen may be performed by lifting the whole arm; blinking by tensing the cheek and forehead in addition to the eyelid. Emotionally and intellectually, there is also a tendency to overinvest in the reaction and the preparation for an event. Even when preventing their tic or habit, sufferers may report increased frustration and negative anticipation. The person may volunteer benefits such as: being seen as efficient, not wasting time, always being on the go, not wasting time, keeping alert.

In other exercises clients can be asked to test efficacy through behavioral experiments and report how this new style feels and functions if they invest less effort. Are they more alert, more able to focus on the goal of the task and keep it simple rather than being clogged up with unnecessary detail or diversions? These benefits are usually illusory and generally the styles of action impede progress rather than accelerate it.

This point can be illustrated by experience exercises. Ask the client to try performing three tasks instead of five tasks in order to experience the greater feeling of accomplishment with fewer tasks. In other exercises the client can be asked to monitor effort during the tasks and relax redundant muscles.

Ask the client to try this exercise: take a typical day where the client may plan to do five jobs. How does the client feel about this? Now plan to do two jobs. Does the client feel better? List the pros and cons of each strategy. Identify where in daily living the client tries to do too much. Invite the client to try performing fewer tasks on at least a couple of days during the week. Don't hesitate to plan these tasks and agree on the days and to invite the client to report on what he or she noticed at the next session.

Through this analysis, it should become apparent to the client that planning to do too much and trying to do too much are highly inefficient and set the client up for failure. A thinking part driving these styles of action is more pervasive in dictating how the client approaches and plans action and feels about the action.

Thoughts associated with Styles of Action: Perfectionism in Personal Standards and Personal Organization

Usually, the thoughts behind the style of planning appear to be in the service of perfectionist goals and are often present with rigid rules and beliefs about the self—such as "Either I do everything at once or I'm lazy," "People will not tolerate me if I'm a little late," or "I may be inadequate and if I don't act as quickly as possible, everyone will know I can't perform." The two types of perfectionism relevant to people with tics and habits are perfectionism about personal standards and personal organization. That is, excessive concern over appearance and excessive concern over the way actions are planned and organized. We give examples of common beliefs associated with each style of action in Table 8.4.

Along with this perfectionism about appearance goes fear of being judged badly by others. Acute awareness of potentially negative judgments regarding tics or habits can lead people with tics or habits to attempt to suppress, delay, or disguise their tics or habits, often with a view to hiding them from others. As already noted these strategies commonly result in increased muscular tension and thus a renewed impetus to tic or habit. There may be attempts to escape or avoid certain emotions because the person cannot deal with them or is trying to fight them (see Table 8.5). Perfectionist standards feed a heightened focus on self, personal appearance (including how one is perceived by others), and bodily proprioceptive sensations (checking if one is feeling "just right"). These processes ultimately feed motor activation and could produce a ceiling level of motor activation). This ceiling effect, due to chronic overactivation, could lead to problems in short-term arousal regulation. This may lead to the difficulties in optimally adapting arousal/activation level to task demand outlined above. As proprioceptive information more often than not indicates tension, effort is more often down-regulated by abandoning tasks than by taking in information from the broad range of sources. If the client relies on feelings of just right to know a task is completed rather than visual cues, we advise they monitor this tendency in Table 8.5. The perfectionist trait might also mean that people feel

Table 8.4 Belief behind styles of actions

————————————————

————————————————

————————————————

————————————————

————————————————

————————————————

Examples of beliefs:

I must always meet high standards in my performance

I must always appear efficient

I must present an unblemished image to the world

Others will judge me badly if I appear too relaxed

You must always be occupied to show you are not slacking

I don't deserve to take it easy

If I'm off guard the worst could happen

I must be vigilant all the time to avoid accidents

You need to keep your mind active to stay alert

If I'm not tensed up I could lose it

If I don't talk quickly people will lose interest in me

I feel I don't have the right to relax for a moment

Table 8.5 Form to check reliance on muscle feedback instead of visual feedback

Today ———————————————

I did not rely on my feelings to accomplish a task

Instead I relied on my senses and visual cues as feedback on performance

they should be in absolute control of sensations, movements, and reactions, which as we noted earlier even if it were possible is counterproductive. So thoughts and beliefs about how to act may be sabotaging a person's movements. We deal in the next chapter specifically with how avoiding emotions, acting on thoughts literally, and fusing too strongly with thoughts dominate preparation (see Table 8.6).

Table 8.6 Thoughts associated with styles of action

Personal styles of action	Feelings	Thoughts

Planning to do less

A perfectionistic and negatively self-focused thinking "style" combines with heightened sensory-motor activation, which it feeds, as people who believe they must always be on the go and invest more effort than necessary are more likely to maintain muscular tension in readiness for the next action. Meanwhile, the over-planning and sense of having to do many things at once make it difficult to be present in the task at hand, which in turn makes it difficult to modulate arousal, perceive, and respond to proprioceptive feedback. The box may be lighter than at first imagined, but that can be hard to notice when one's mind is busy antici-pating the next action. In addition, chronic feelings of frustration and impatience may distract attentional resources away from sensory information. This leads to muscles staying in a chronic state of heightened tension, which in turn can feed and be fed by hypervigilance to sensory state. In contexts where heightened ten-sion is a risk, such as a performance or social appraisal, ticking, as a temporary way to release tension becomes highly likely. But tension obviously impedes relaxation mentally and physically. Ask the client to refer back to Table 8.1, which lists personal style of action and indicate how he or she will plan less.

To experience this link, lie down or in a comfortable chair and bring some pleasant thoughts to mind, perhaps a pleasant memory, and notice the feelings. Now tense the body as much as possible and attempt to bring to mind the same pleasant memory. Notice the feelings now. Chances are it was harder to contact pleasant feelings in the second condition, illustrating the impact of muscle ten-sion on feelings.

One of the keys to treating tics or habits effectively is to help clients do less and plan to do less. This reduces what occasions tension in the first place and will in turn increase effectiveness and life satisfaction. This converting of the rigidity of thinking into flexibility and adaptability of thoughts driving styles of action can be applied to all perfectionist beliefs about acting, and some examples are given in Table 8.8 and Table 8.9. In Table 8.7, we ask the client to practice the thought flexibility.

Table 8.7 Thought flexibility; testing alternative thoughts

Situation:_____

Habitual thinking	Reality check	More constructive thinking

Table 8.8 Thought flexibility; testing alternative thoughts in a social professional meeting

Situation: Social professional meeting

Habitual thinking	Reality check	More constructive thinking
I would have nothing interesting to say	Why do I think that I wouldn't have anything interesting to say since such meetings have gone well in the past?	In such situations, I am able to maintain the conversation. The worst that could happen would be that the interlocutor looks away toward someone else
I must properly represent my service	Will the other person base their idea of the entirety of my service on this one meeting?	I try to represent my service as well as possible, but others wouldn't base their idea of my service solely on our conversation. I don't necessarily have to know everything; I can redirect a person toward the right resources
They are going to think I am incompetent	Do I base my judgement of the competence of a person on one meeting? Why would others do it?	
It is up to me to fill in the silences	If there are silences, aren't the others just as responsible for these silences.	The others are as much responsible as me for the silence
I am afraid to look silly	If I end up looking ridiculous, would it be so catastrophic?	Instead of worrying about what others think of me, I should reverse this thought to ask what I think of them

Table 8.9 Thought flexibility; testing alternative thoughts when preparing for a conference

Situation: <u>Prepare conference</u>

Habitual thinking	Emotion	Reality check	More constructive thinking
- This conference must be excellent, everything must be perfect	Apprehension	What would happen if everything wasn't perfect?	This conference must be well prepared, but it doesn't need to be absolutely perfect. It is important, but it is not the most important conference I have ever given (the importance of relativizing)
- I would like for the others not only to find this conference good—I would love for them to be really impressed	Inquietude	The audience would still be most likely satisfied, they are not expecting perfection	By pacing my efforts and by avoiding putting in more energy and tension than necessary, I will be more efficient (I will have more energy left) for my other tasks
- Everything I do must be of quality	Fatigue	Is it truly necessary that the audience are impressed if they had a good time nonetheless? No.	
- The others will be disappointed if the conference is not up to par	Depressed	Regarding this concern to be up to the task, are those expectations coming from others or myself? Most of the time, it is from myself	Up to a certain point, putting in supplementary effort would bring only few additional results
- If I don't put in a lot of time and energy, it's not going to be good	Stressed		
- I prefer to do as much as possible myself (though there are two of us) so that the conference corresponds to my quality criteria.	Worry	Is this conference really worth all the effort (tension, less sleeping time, etc.)	By sharing the work burden, it is possible that the work wouldn't have ended up as I wanted to, but it is possible that my other coworkers would shred a new light on the matter, bringing new ideas that would make the conference better
- I have to be able to fulfil the ideal that I have in mind. I must do everything perfectly to balance with my lack of confidence in myself	Frustrated	This conference is worth being well prepared, but not to the point of jeopardizing my health	I have the capacity, but I choose to stop

In this chapter, we have looked at specific thoughts and emotions behind problematic styles of planning and action. Next, in Chapters 10 and 11, we'll look at effective ways to work with unhelpful thoughts patterns and the emotional aspects of tic and habit disorders.

Therapist checklist for styles of action

Client has identified key styles of action relevant to them personally	Yes / No ❏ ❏
Client has attempted the behavioral cost exercise to illustrate behavioral ineffectiveness of: overinvestment, overactivity, overpreparation	Yes / No ❏ ❏
Client understands how styles of action contribute to stress and tension	Yes / No ❏ ❏
Client identifies perfectionist thoughts and beliefs as the source of unhelpful styles of action	Yes / No ❏ ❏
Client plans to do less and cites concrete examples	Yes / No ❏ ❏
Client has attempted behavioral experiments of preparing and planning less activities, being more flexible and producing less tension.	Yes / No ❏ ❏

9

Experiential Avoidance, Cognitive Fusion, and the Matrix

In this chapter we discuss the important role of experiential avoidance and cognitive fusion in perpetuating tension, how the acceptance and commitment therapy (ACT) matrix can serve as a tool to improve flow, how to tell the difference between inner experience and five-senses experience, and finally how all this knowledge can be integrated into changing the style of action by use of the ACT matrix.

Experiential Avoidance and Cognitive Fusion

Experiential avoidance and cognitive fusion are two main contributors to psychopathology (Hayes et al., 2012). Experiential avoidance refers to the natural tendency humans have to escape, avoid, or somehow modify the advent, frequency, or intensity of particular experiential states: feelings, emotions, or bodily sensations. Cognitive fusion refers to a tendency to take one's thoughts literally and confuse thoughts and their content for the experience they symbolize as if thoughts, history, and self-conceptions were fused to the person and their way of perceiving the world. Metaphorically speaking, cognitive fusion is taking the map for the territory.

Experiential avoidance as measured by the Acceptance and Action Questionnaire (AAQ-II, Bond et al., 2011) in Table 9.1 and Table 9.2 has been identified as a transdiagnostic pathological process. In measures the extend to which the client escapes from experience. It has been found to be associated with a broad range of negative mental and physical health outcomes. Reductions in experiential avoidance have been found to be a major contributor to clinical improvements. Further, experiential avoidance has been found to impact the effectiveness of coping strategies, emotion regulation, and cognitive reappraisal. Although experiential avoidance has not been studied in relation to tics and Tourette's, its role in trichotillomania and skin picking has been researched. Similar dysfunctional cognitions and negative affects have been identified for habit disorders and for tics or habits, and been linked to disorder severity. In trichotillomania, experiential avoidance may account for the link between negative affect, dysfunctional cognitions, and disorder severity (Norberg, Wetterneck,

Managing Tic and Habit Disorders: A Cognitive Psychophysiological Approach with Acceptance Strategies, First Edition. Kieron P O'Connor, Marc E Lavoie, and Benjamin Schoendorff.
© 2017 John Wiley & Sons, Ltd. Published 2017 by John Wiley & Sons, Ltd.
Companion Website: www.wiley.com/go/oconnor/managingticandhabitdsorders

Table 9.1 Acceptance and Action Questionnaire–II (AAQ-II) (Bond et al., 2011)

Below you will find a list of statements. Please rate how true each statement is for you by circling a number next to it. Use the scale below to make your choice.

1	2	3	4	5	6	7
Never true	Very seldom true	Seldom true	Sometimes true	Frequently true	Almost always true	Always true

	1	2	3	4	5	6	7
1. My painful experiences and memories make it difficult for me to live a life that I would value	1	2	3	4	5	6	7
2. I'm afraid of my feelings	1	2	3	4	5	6	7
3. I worry about not being able to control my worries and feelings	1	2	3	4	5	6	7
4. My painful memories prevent me from having a fulfilling life	1	2	3	4	5	6	7
5. Emotions cause problems in my life	1	2	3	4	5	6	7
6. It seems like most people are handling their lives better than I am	1	2	3	4	5	6	7
7. Worries get in the way of my success	1	2	3	4	5	6	7

Note: This is a one-factor measure of psychological inflexibility, or experiential avoidance. Score the scale by summing the seven items. Higher scores equal greater levels of psychological inflexibility.

Table 9.2 Tics and Habits Acceptance and Action Questionnaire (THAAQ)

Directions: Below you will find a list of statements. Please rate the truth of each statement as it applies to you. Use the following rating scale to make your choices. For instance, if you believe a statement is "Always true," you would write a 7 next to that statement.

Never true	Very seldom true	Seldom true	Sometimes true	Frequently true	Almost always true	Always true
1	2	3	4	5	6	7

_____ 1. My tics or habits make it difficult for me to live a life that I value
_____ 2. I care too much about my tics or habits
_____ 3. I shut down when I feel bad about my tics or habits
_____ 4. My tics or habits must change before I can take important steps in my life
_____ 5. Worrying about my tics or habits takes up too much of my time
_____ 6. If I start to think about my tics or habits, I try to think about something else
_____ 7. Before I can make any serious plans, I have to feel better about my tics or habits
_____ 8. I will have better control over my life if I can control my negative thoughts and feelings about my tics or habits
_____ 9. My tics or habits make me a different person
_____ 10. My tics and habits cause problems in my life
_____ 11. When I start thinking about my tics or habits, it's hard to do anything else
_____ 12. I avoid certain activities or situations because of my tics

Woods, & Conelea, 2007). In people with tic or habit disorder, wanting things to feel "just right" is one of the many forms experiential avoidance can take; having trouble tolerating frustration and irritation is another one. People with tic or habit disorder are often trying to say or not say different messages at the same time. They may be trying to be polite and in a hurry at the same time. They may want to say a word or carry out an action but at the same time feel inhibited and end up repressing or avoiding their feelings.

Cognitive fusion also plays a part. People with a tic or habit disorder might be highly fused with thoughts about how they look to others, how abnormal they are, and more generally with thoughts about how things should be. Many of the thoughts motivating the overcomplicating and overplanning styles of action, discussed earlier, may be taken literally (doing less really means I'm lazy), and contribute to maintaining tics or habits. Cognitive fusion is associated with anxiety and depression, health anxiety, and body dissatisfaction. It can interact with experiential avoidance in predicting depression and anxiety. Cognitive fusion can be measured by the Cognitive Fusion Questionnaire, the CFQ (Gillanders et al., 2014, Table 9.3).

Training acceptance, the ability to be with one's experience without undue defense, can contribute to deepening your clinical work with tic disorder clients. Similarly, helping clients to defuse from sticky thoughts can help them adopt more workable styles of planning.

Table 9.3 Cognitive Fusion Questionnaire (CFQ) (Gillanders et al., 2014)

1 Never true	2 Very seldom true	3 Seldom true	4 Sometimes true	5 Frequently true	6 Almost always true	7 Always true
1. My thoughts causes me distress or emotional pain				1	2	3	4	5	6	7
2. I get so caught up in my thoughts that I am unable to do the things that I most want to do				1	2	3	4	5	6	7
3. I overanalyze situations to the point where it's unhelpful to me				1	2	3	4	5	6	7
4. I struggle with my thoughts				1	2	3	4	5	6	7
5. I get upset with myself for having certain thoughts				1	2	3	4	5	6	7
6. I tend to get very entangled in my thoughts				1	2	3	4	5	6	7
7. It's such a struggle to let go of upsetting thoughts even when I know that letting go would be helpful				1	2	3	4	5	6	7

Improving Flow and Goal Directed Action Using the ACT Matrix

The ACT matrix is a diagram that can serve to increase client engagement in therapy as well as prepare clients for acceptance and defusion work.

The matrix diagram is composed of two perpendicular lines. One is a horizontal line representing a discrimination between actions engaged to move away from (or under the control of) unwanted thoughts and feelings and actions engaged to move toward who or what is important (values). The vertical line represents the discrimination between five-senses experience—what can be perceived through one's eyes, ears, nose, taste, or sense of touch—and inner or mental experience—thoughts, feelings, memories, and bodily sensations (including proprioception). As the two lines intersect, they map out four quadrants. Clients are invited to sort their experiences in the two lower quadrants and their behavior in the two upper quadrants (see Figures 9.1 and 9.2). As our treatment for tics or habits includes training in discrimination between high risk and low risk contexts for ticking as well as discrimination between tension and relaxation in particular muscle groups, you can also introduce the matrix as a tool for further discrimination training.

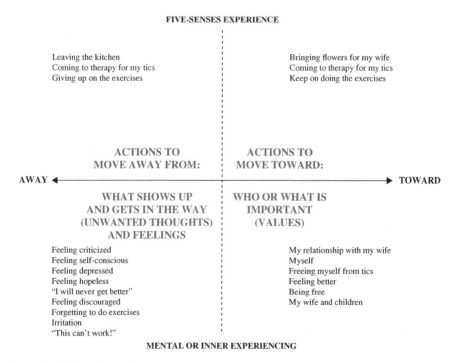

Figure 9.1 The ACT matrix example

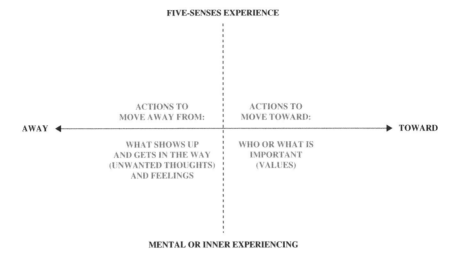

Figure 9.2 The ACT matrix

You may choose to introduce the ACT matrix at any time during treatment. The dialogue below illustrates how the matrix can be introduced to clients consulting for tics or habits disorders.

T: Before we move to looking in some more detail at your experience with tics (or a specific habit disorder), can I show you a point of view that many people have found helpful to do what's important to them, even in the presence of obstacles? In learning an effective way to reduce your tics, there is a good chance that you will come across such obstacles and this point of view may help you successfully overcome them.

C: Okay.

T: [Draws two perpendicular lines with arrows pointing to the left and right of the horizontal line on a piece of paper]. The horizontal line represents the difference between what we do to move away from what we don't want to think or feel, like fear, irritation, or stress, here on the left, and what we do to move toward who or what is important to us in life. So I write "away" on the left and "toward" on the right. Can you remember ever doing something to move away from some difficult thought or feeling?

C: Yes, only yesterday I left the kitchen when I felt criticized by my wife.

T: Excellent! So leaving the kitchen would go up here top left and feeling criticized would go bottom left. And can you remember ever doing something to move toward someone or something important to you?

C: Yes, for example, buying flowers for my wife's birthday, and also coming to see you for help with my tics.

T: Excellent. So buying flowers for your wife's birthday and coming to see me for help with tics go top right. And who or what is important to you in doing this?

C: Well, my wife, my relationship with her. And about coming here?
I guess myself, freeing myself from the tics and all the grief they have
caused me.

T: Do I hear that there is also an "away" part in coming here? Perhaps
away from the consequences of the tics?

C: Oh yes, I feel really self-conscious about them, and depressed.
Sometimes I feel hopeless, that I will never get better.

T: Oh so feeling self-conscious, depressed, and hopeless, and the
thought "I will never get better" may be things you'd like to move away
from?

C: You bet!

T: Okay good, so we can write them bottom left. And coming to therapy
in the top left as well as in the top right. So basically this is the point of
view. Let's see if there are more things you can see through it right now.
Who or what is important in your coming here to treat your tics?

C: Me, feeling better, being free, my wife and children also because
I keep on thinking this has an impact on them.

T: Good. Let me write all this in the bottom right. Now can I ask you, if
you could choose between two lives, one in which most—but not all—of
what you do is to move away from this bottom left stuff and another life in
which what you do is more often about moving toward the people or
things that are important to you, which of these two lives would you
choose?

C: The one on the right of course!

T: Great, because me too! And our work is going to be about helping
you choose the life on the right, and specifically, teaching you how to
more easily choose to do these things up here on the right, even in the
presence of stuff showing up down here on the left. Now back to tics. I am
going to introduce you to an approach that has been shown to work to
help you bring your tics under control. It will take work and dedication,
but there is a good chance you'll succeed. Where would you put using this
approach in this diagram?

C: Top right I guess.

T: Excellent. But let me tell you something. As you start applying the
method I will show you, stuff may show up bottom left and get in the way.
Any idea what this could be?

C: Well I can easily get discouraged. And I can forget do things if I have
too much to do.

T: Exactly! Maybe feeling discouraged will show up; maybe forgetful-
ness. Maybe irritation, maybe thoughts that it can't work or that it does
not make sense, or does not go fast enough, to name a few common inner
obstacles people with tics have noticed. And if these obstacles show up to
tell you to stop using the approach, I wonder what the person you want to
be would do?

C: Ideally, stick with doing things up here on the right? But do you think
it will work?

T: As I say, there is a good chance it can work. Now let's look more closely at the situations in which your tics show up and what these different situations have in common. You see there could be similarities up here, in what you can see around you, in places or situations. And there could be similarities down there, in what you think and how you feel. As we progress with our work, we'll explore how you can more easily recognize different situations and what you can do to better control your ticking.

In this extract, the client was introduced to the ACT matrix in a participatory way. Rather than explaining the model to the client, the therapist gently guides the client through an exploration of the point of view, setting the stage for the next step: identifying the diverse contexts in which tics or habits take place and those in which ticking is reduced.

Discriminating Thoughts, Actions, and Experiences

Once the client has been introduced to—and practiced—the discrimination between relaxed and tense muscular tone, the therapist can invite him or her to practice discriminating between five-senses experience and inner or mental experience. This discrimination will serve the client well in learning how to reconnect action planning with sensory information rather than the excessive reliance on waiting to feel "just right" that feeds ticking, or that they have done enough or been active enough. Further, the link between thoughts, emotions, and action can be further explored by showing how the mind tends to respond to thoughts and emotions as if they were things happening in the physical world, which can easily trigger premotor activation and muscular tension. Through a simple discrimination exercise, the client can learn to unlink thoughts and emotions from muscular tension.

The dialogue below illustrates how to introduce this.

T: You know our minds are our greatest tools. Over millennia, they have allowed us to learn to control a lot of what goes on in the world outside our skin. Look around us. There is very little we can see that has not been modified, controlled in some way—thanks to our human intelligence. Furniture, climate control, gardens, means of transportation. As a species, we have unparalleled abilities to control the world around us, the world of five-senses experience. Is it any wonder that, when our minds turn toward the world of inner experience and see things they don't like, such as uncomfortable thoughts and feelings, they should try to control them? But does it work?

C: What do you mean?

T: Well, how many times, over the past week, have you thought of a pink unicorn?

C: None.

T: Good, so now for the next 30 s, whatever you do, just make sure that you don't think of either a pink unicorn or anything that makes you think of one. This is not about performing or proving anything to me, it's about noticing what shows up for you. Okay?

C: Okay I'll try.

T: Time's up. What did you notice?

C: The more I tried not to think of the unicorn, the more I thought of it.

T: Right, and yet, have you ever noticed your mind telling you not to think of something?

C: Sure. All the time.

T: What chance have we got? But you know what's weird? It's as if our minds couldn't get it and they will again and again tell us not to think of something. As a matter of fact, sometimes we can, but it's a lot like holding a ball underwater. The bigger the ball, the harder it is and the bigger the splash when we let go. And you know? Maybe it's not so different for feelings. Imagine that I hooked you up to a lie detector. These actually detect changes in skin conductance and blood pressure caused by stress and anxiety. Imagine that I now put a gun to your head and told you I'd shoot at the slightest sign of stress. How long do you think you'd survive?

C: Not long... Seconds?

T: Seconds, right! And how often do you notice your mind going: "Don't stress, don't feel any anxiety, it's really important! It's vital!"

C: Often enough.

T: Exactly, what chance have we got? And again it's as if our minds can't see this, no matter how smart they are. It's as if there were two different rules, one for the world of five-senses experience, the world outside the skin, and one for the world inside the skin. Outside the skin, the rule that works is something like: *If you don't like it, think about it, try different things and you'll finally come to control it.* But for the world inside the skin, the world of inner experience, maybe the rule is more something like: *The more you try to control it, the more...*

C: you're stuck with it?

T: Exactly, the more you're stuck with it. You see the problem is our minds have trouble noticing the difference between five-senses and inner experience in a way similar to your initial difficulties in noticing the difference between tension and relaxation. When you can't notice the difference between five-senses experience and inner experience, the danger is you will instinctively respond to inner experience by tensing your muscles in preparation for action. In the world of five senses, it makes a lot of sense. You see a wolf, you prepare for action so you can survive. But in the world of inner experience, you think of a wolf or simply feel some irritation, and you respond by tensing your muscles. That doesn't help you in any way, but it feeds the tension and your urges to tic. So right now, we're going to practice noticing the difference between five-senses and inner experience so it becomes easier for you to discriminate and not tense when some inner experience shows up. Okay?

C: Okay.

T: So let me prepare some cards. On this one I'll write "5 Senses" and on that one "Inner/Mental." I'll also make a couple for me. Now we're going to practice sorting between five-senses and mental experience by simply noticing whatever experience shows up for us moment to moment and raise the card that best corresponds to our experience of the moment. I'll do it with you so we both get to look stupid, Okay?

C: Okay.

T: Just to be clear: five-senses experience means something that comes to you through one of your five senses: something you can see, hear, smell, taste, or some touch sensation on your skin. Everything else is mental or inner experience: thoughts, emotions, mental images, and also inner bodily sensations, such as pain, urges, or whatever feelings show up inside the skin that are not caused by the touch of some object. In other words, if it does not show up through one of your five senses, then it's mental or inner experience. Now before we start, let me alert you to some common experiences when first practicing this exercise. Experiences such as "What is the point of this exercise?" What kind of experience is this?

C: Mental?

T: Yes mental! Experiences such as: "We look stupid" or urges to laugh. What kind of experiences are these?

C: Mental?

T: Good, and also experiences such as: "I don't know what kind of experience I'm having right now." What kind of experience is that?

C: Mental.

T: You're getting good at this. So now if you've got it, at any moment in time, we both should have at least one card held up, right? So let's practice for 1 min.

At the end of the assigned minute, ask the client for feedback. Some clients will have noticed more mental experience, some clients both mental and five senses in rapid succession, some clients will have noticed both kinds of experiences showing up at the same time. Whatever the client says, validate it by saying something like: "You noticed that, well noticed." If the client has noticed both five-senses and mental experience showing up at the same time, ask if they could still notice the difference between the two.

Next tell your client this exercise is like a stretching exercise that can help them not get caught into interacting with inner or mental experience as if it were five-senses experience. It can help them not tense up or release tension when particular thoughts or feelings show up. For people with tics or habits, interacting with inner experience, whether beliefs, anticipations, or impulses to act, as though it is five-senses experience leads to tensing up unnecessarily and feeds the tic and habit loops. Invite the client to practice this exercise at least 1 min per day every day and tell them you'll debrief on what they have noticed when you next meet. You can also use the matrix and point to the vertical line to help your client notice the difference between five-senses and mental or inner experience. Using the matrix has the advantage of training your client in seeing toward and away behavior as that which can be controlled, and inner experience, whether aversive or appetitive, as that which can not so easily be controlled (see Table 9.4).

Table 9.4 Distinguishing inner and five-senses experience

Date/hour	Internal thoughts/experiences	Five-senses experiences

Date/hour	Internal thoughts/experiences	Five-senses experiences

Using the ACT Matrix to Work with Styles of Action

The ACT matrix can be an effective complementary tool to help increase flexibility of styles of planning and action. The styles of planning and action that promote tension and the tic or habit loops are: doing too much at once; not taking time to relax; doing things too quickly; seeking perfection in small things; hiding one's feelings; and adopting tense body postures. Sorting these in the matrix can help clients identify what maintains these styles of action. Using the matrix, the client can write these actions top left, as moves away or under the control of unwanted inner experience. Invite your clients to describe how these styles of action might apply to them, and what they can be seen doing (as if they were being filmed on some reality TV show) when they engage in these styles of action. Next invite your clients to identify what inner experience shows up that gets them to engage in these actions. It's best to let the client identify what can drive these actions. Common experiences will be stress, feeling one has to perform, fear of judgment, fear of rejection if one isn't perfect, and so on. Write these down in the bottom left of the matrix (see Figures 9.1 and 9.2).

Next tell your clients that all these things that show up bottom left can hook us into behaving differently than we would have had we not gotten hooked by them, in pretty much the same way that, when they bite hooks, fish get pulled in a direction that they would not have swum in had they not gotten hooked. Ask your client what fish would do if they could notice that hooks are hooks. Would they need in any way to get rid of hooks? Would they need to understand or explain hooks? Would they need to change hooks in any way? If they could notice that hooks are hooks, fish would not need to do anything with hooks other than simply swim around them. The same can be true of us. By practicing noticing our hooks and what we do next, we can gradually come to recognize them and bite less or even notice when we do bite and then flail less against the hook. This last point is particularly important for clients with tic and habit disorders, as struggling once hooked will likely lead to more tension. Our inability to notice the difference between five-senses and mental experience will easily get us hooked. Confusing the two naturally leads to us trying to react to inner experience with some action and thus premotor activation (see Figure 9.3).

These styles of action apply both to tics and habits, but in habits the way emotions are detected and regulated in everyday life is important as well.

HOOKS WORKSHEET Write your hooks on the bait, and on the fishing line, write what you do next. For example you might write "Anger" on a worm, then write "Raise my voice and leave" on the line.

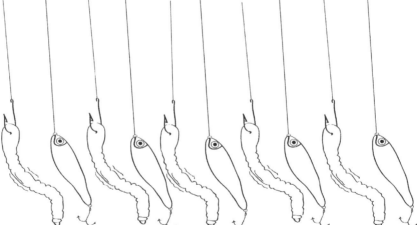

Figure 9.3 Hooks worksheet

Therapist checklist for experiential avoidance and the ACT matrix

The client understands experiential avoidance and valued action (i.e., the difference between away and toward moves)	Yes / No ❏ ❏
The client is able to list examples related to tics or habits	Yes / No ❏ ❏
The client understands the role of cognitive fusion in their tic or habit onset and gives examples (i.e., is able to identify hooks and what they do next)	Yes / No ❏ ❏
The client relates the ACT matrix to tic or habit behaviors	Yes / No ❏ ❏
The client can apply the ACT matrix to their styles of action	Yes / No ❏ ❏

10

Emotional Regulation and Overcoming
the Habit–Shame Loop

Although perfectionist styles of action are relevant to both tics and habits, other emotions such as feelings of depression, worthlessness, lack of self-satisfaction, and frustration can trigger tics or habits.

In this chapter we round up our discussion of flexibility by addressing emotional flexibility in the control of the client's tic or habit onset: how to identify trigger emotions and cope with them adaptively. Negative emotions and rumination can lead to excessive self-criticism, and feelings of shame and guilt.

Patterns of talking and thinking can contribute to the client's feelings of guilt and shame about him or herself and his or her actions, and so we encourage the client to learn how not to become a prisoner of his or her own self-talk and fixed way of feeling and thinking about his or her actions. In so doing, we look at the stories the client tells about him or herself about who he or she is and what he or she can do and encourage him or her to base these on his or her real self and not stale beliefs and metaphors.

Emotions

Emotions are an integral part of the tic and habit cycles. Research has shown that habits such as hair pulling, skin picking, and nail biting, although they cause distress, are also maintained as they provide relief from tension and negative emotions. They are a form of experiential avoidance with the positive function of regulating emotions, which encourage a destructive loop. One researcher suggested that people pull their hair when they're both over- and understimulated (Penzel, 1995). Clients with habits typically experience a broader range of negative emotions and more difficulty in regulating them than clients with tics. But tics can also be triggered by diverse emotions. For example, for one client tic onset occurred when he experienced shame, and another person experienced onset when he heard awkward political speeches that made him cringe.

So the emotions associated with tics or habits tend to be dominated by frustration, impatience, and dissatisfaction derived largely from a perfectionist style of organization and planning as noted earlier, but more complex emotions of shame might also be present, especially in public. However, triggers and relief may stem from frustration and impatience more than any other emotions (see Figure 10.1).

Managing Tic and Habit Disorders: A Cognitive Psychophysiological Approach with Acceptance Strategies, First Edition. Kieron P O'Connor, Marc E Lavoie, and Benjamin Schoendorff.
© 2017 John Wiley & Sons, Ltd. Published 2017 by John Wiley & Sons, Ltd.
Companion Website: www.wiley.com/go/oconnor/managingticandhabitdsorders

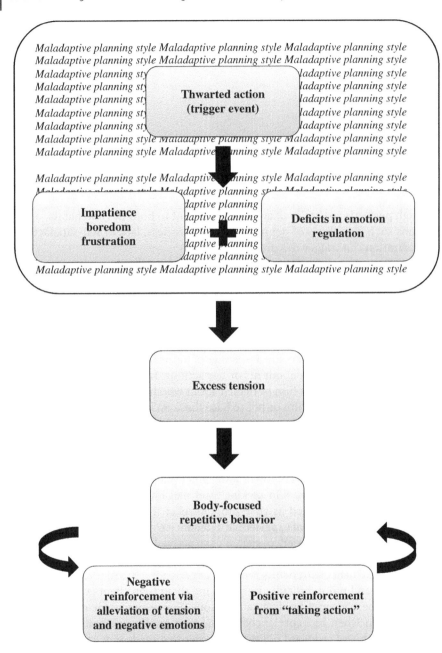

Figure 10.1 Frustration/action triggers for habit disorders

Habit disorders tend to be associated with complex emotion regulation (Robert, O'Connor, Aardema & Bélanger, 2015; Robert, O'Connor & Bélanger, 2015).

For people with tics or habits, uncomfortable emotions are commonly a result of ineffective action preparation strategies, such as preparing for two conflicting tasks at the same time, either within the same task or in different tasks. The aim is to help clients become more fully aware of their emotions and their physical reactions to them, and adopt effective strategies to makes space for whatever they are feeling without undue tension.

In clinical practice, it can be useful to evaluate clients on three dimensions:

1) Ability to identify emotions.
2) Ability to cope constructively with negative emotions rather than getting hooked by them.
3) Ability to accept emotions and reduce their negative impact on behavior.

We provide evaluation forms in Tables 10.1–10.3.

In addition, people with habit disorders might show evidence of difficulties in regulating emotions, as well as highly negative self-perceptions and critical self-talk.

The forms are self-explanatory and highlight problems the client may have in dealing with beliefs, worrying about beliefs, worrying about control, dealing with the inevitability of being overwhelmed by emotions, dealing with certain emotions, avoidance of feelings, reacting to emotions, accepting emotions, judging emotions, and snapping out of emotions. A high score on any of these emotional dimensions can be discussed and elaborated on with the client. An emotional problem, but if the client carries out our exercises this will help.

Table 10.1 Self-criticism Self-judgment Questionnaire

I always criticize myself	Yes / No ❏ ❏
I'm never good enough	Yes / No ❏ ❏
Other people see me as a failure	Yes / No ❏ ❏
I often make the wrong choices	Yes / No ❏ ❏
I'm ashamed of my actions	Yes / No ❏ ❏
My performance sucks	Yes / No ❏ ❏
I should be more competent	Yes / No ❏ ❏
After each task, I start questioning myself	Yes / No ❏ ❏

Table 10.2 Difficulties in Emotion Regulation Scale (DERS) (adapted from Gratz & Roemer, 2004)

Please indicate how often the following statements apply to you by writing the appropriate number from the scale below on the line beside each item:

1	2	3	4	5
Almost never	Sometimes	About half the time	Most of the time	Almost always
(0–10%)	(11–33%)	(36–65%)	(66–90%)	(91–100%)

_____ 1) I pay attention to how I feel (A)

_____ 2) I experience my emotions as overwhelming and out of control (L)

_____ 3) I have no idea how I am feeling (C)

_____ 4) I have difficulty making sense out of my feelings (C)

_____ 5) I am attentive to my feelings (A)

_____ 6) When I'm upset, I become embarrassed for feeling that way (N)

_____ 7) When I'm upset, I become out of control (L)

_____ 8) When I'm upset,I believe that I'll end up feeling very depressed (P)

_____ 9) When I'm upset, I have difficulty focusing on other things (D)

_____ 10) When I'm upset, I feel ashamed with myself for feeling that way (N)

_____ 11) When I'm upset, I feel guilty for feeling that way (N)

_____ 12) When I'm upset, I have difficulty concentrating (D)

_____ 13) When I'm upset, I have difficulty controlling my behaviors (L)

_____ 14) When I'm upset, I believe there is nothing I can do to make myself feel better (P)

_____ 15) When I'm upset, I become irritated with myself for feeling that way (N)

_____ 16) When I'm upset, it takes me a long time to feel better (P)

Note: This questionnaire measure six elements in your reactions to emotions:

(1) N= non-acceptance of emotional responses; (2) D= difficulties engaging in goal directed behavior; (3) L= loss of control over feelings; (4) A= awareness of feelings; (5) P= poor emotional regulation; and (6) C= clarity of emotions.

Table 10.3 Affective Regulation Scale (ARS) (Shusterman, Feld, Baer, & Keuthen, 2009)

Name: _____ Date: _____

Below you will see a list of moods. Please check the circle that indicates your ability to control each of these moods. How easily can you "snap out of it"?

	Never able to control	Rarely able to control	Can control about half the time	Can control most of the time	Always able to control
Bored	❏	❏	❏	❏	❏
Angry	❏	❏	❏	❏	❏
Guilty	❏	❏	❏	❏	❏
Indifferent	❏	❏	❏	❏	❏
Tense	❏	❏	❏	❏	❏

Table 10.3 (Continued)

	Never able to control	Rarely able to control	Can control about half the time	Can control most of the time	Always able to control
Irritable	❏	❏	❏	❏	❏
Sad	❏	❏	❏	❏	❏
Anxious	❏	❏	❏	❏	❏
Ashamed	❏	❏	❏	❏	❏
Afraid	❏	❏	❏	❏	❏
Dissatisfied	❏	❏	❏	❏	❏
Frustrated	❏	❏	❏	❏	❏
Preoccupied	❏	❏	❏	❏	❏

Please indicate how likely each mood is to cause hair pulling, skin picking, or nail biting.

	Never	Sometimes	Often
Bored	❏	❏	❏
Angry	❏	❏	❏
Guilty	❏	❏	❏
Indifferent	❏	❏	❏
Tense	❏	❏	❏
Irritable	❏	❏	❏
Sad	❏	❏	❏
Anxious	❏	❏	❏
Afraid	❏	❏	❏
Dissatisfied	❏	❏	❏
Frustrated			
Preoccupied	❏	❏	❏

The Habit–Shame Loop

People with habit disorders, and to a lesser extent, tics, tend to get stuck in ineffective emotional regulation loops. They engage in the habit to relieve unwanted emotion such as feelings of boredom, frustration, tension, and including feelings of inactivity. Indeed, hair pullers and skin pickers report decreases in boredom, tension, and anxiety post-pulling. But then they experience guilt, shame, and sadness. People will typically pull their hair when they feel down. Those negative affects can in turn feed frustration and tension, and further feed the loop. As our research suggests, people with habit disorders find it hard to snap out of difficult emotions.

Some people gain stimulation from the habit. It is a mild form of self-mutilation and may have aspects in common with self-harm, and some people may feel more alive with the sensation, particularly if they already have trouble living with and identifying normal feelings and sensations. Hair pulling or skin picking is a little like smoking: it can produce stimulation and calm the client down depending on context. Unfortunately, it also produces a close cycle for rumination whilst pulling and hence maintains low mood and recriminations.

Examine with the client what specific emotion they have difficulty in identifying or regulating. Find out the thought behind the emotion and whether it is flexible and, if not, how it can become flexible with the technique already noted in Chapter 8.

Variants of perfectionism may drive the experience of a client not living up to his or her standards and postulating an ideal self which he or she can never live up to, which encourages feelings of worthlessness. People may pull or scratch or bite when they are alone and in a low mood, and may have more problems than normal in snapping out of emotions. All these points indicate difficulties regulating and coping with emotions, a sensitivity to emotions, and a difficulty identifying and engaging in emotions constructively.

Adaptive and Maladaptive Coping

Maladaptive coping strategies for emotional regulation include blame, rumination, self-criticism, reproaches, condemnation, negative self-criticism, and catastrophizing. Self-criticism in particular can feed on rumination. When the brain is idling it is ripe for rumination and pulling aids rumination. Self-criticism can be both internally and externally focused. Internal criticism focuses on feelings of inadequacy and inferiority; external criticism on disgust and shame regarding one's behaviors. Shame can also be internal and external. Internally focused shame is characterized by relentless criticism, devaluation of self, feelings of inadequacy, badness, and oddness or abnormality. Externally focused shame is typified by imagining the condemning, ridiculing, or disgusted thoughts and feelings of others, and the impression of being exposed or discovered or stripped bare in front of others. Self-criticism can easily diverge into self-punishment and auto-mutilation.

People with habit disorders can often consider themselves as worthless, as failures, unable to accomplish tasks competently. Such feelings are fed by self-talk. Here are some descriptions of how people with tic and habits disorders can talk to themselves: "I am such a useless person," "I am so weak I can't stop pulling," "I am a weirdo with my tics or habits," "I am such an idiot for pulling my hair," "When will I ever stop being such a failure?"

We outline below acceptance- and mindfulness-based emotion identification and regulation strategies that are particularly well suited to people with tic and habit disorders.

There are a number of steps in addressing emotional issues and maladaptive coping strategies, including self-talk. They divide broadly into strategies aimed at helping to better identify, name, and accept emotions and strategies aimed at dysfunctional cognitive styles and self-talk. Clients can fill in the two forms given in Table 10.3, which highlight individually emotional difficulties. Emotional regulation breaks down into several components, and by filling in the forms in Tables 10.1–10.3 client and therapist can identify problem emotions and maladaptive coping with and snapping out of the emotions. Client and therapist can then use the strategies outlined in Chapter 5 to identify thoughts and activities associated with the emotions and introduce a more flexible approach.

Making friends with emotions: Identifying and naming emotions

Invite clients to identify what the dominant emotion is in a number of their most salient at-risk situations. You can ask for recent instances of ticking or habit and invite them to describe what they were feeling. If the client is having trouble naming the emotion, offer prompts (but do not implant suggestions), such as: frustration, irritation, sadness, boredom, impatience, shame, guilt, and so on. Once the client has identified an emotion, invite the person to point to a location in the body where the emotion is the most intense (if she is not sure, you can invite the client to point randomly, as gradually her ability to locate emotions will increase). Be gentle and patient as some clients are so detached from their feelings that they might at first struggle with naming and locating emotion. A client may report that she is feeling bored. Next invite her to notice what bodily posture she adopts when this emotion shows up and invite her to relax whatever muscle group she is unnecessarily tensing. Can she notice what the emotion does when she tenses up? Can she notice if it might be easier to receive emotion with more or less tension?

Validating Emotion

Validate that it's perfectly natural to experience a whole range of emotions; that emotions in themselves are not necessarily problematic, although they can be unpleasant—they are an important signal that can be put to good use. Making space for them and learning to observe them with curiosity can help guide our actions. Some emotions such as anger may signal that one feels threatened in some way, and the perception or the emotion can be accepted without directing action. The emotional message can be received, then a workable action planned in the way we feel appropriate. Some clients need coaching in expressing emotions. They might be afraid to express negative emotion or be fused with rules that these should never be expressed. Let them know that expressing emotion is perfectly okay, and that they can still choose how they express their feelings. They may, for example, express that they feel angry, without necessarily speaking in a highly angry tone.

Other emotions might signal that things are unworkable in the way we organize them. For example, the impatience and irritation that come with overactive and overcomplicating action might be a sign that it's time to rethink how the client plans actions.

Clients who experience shame and self-criticism are often fused with unrealistic perfectionist standards about the self (Pélisser & O'Connor, 2004). Helping them uncover these standards and bringing to light their role in feeding self-criticism and non-acceptance can help. Questions such as: "What kind of a person does your mind say you should be?" "Does your mind believe you have a right to make mistakes?" "Does your mind ever allow you to be imperfect?" can be effective. Once these unattainably high standards have been uncovered, suggest they may contribute to tension, to unworkable action styles, and feed the tic and habit loops.

What if the client could accept herself as she is? What if she could look at herself through the eyes of a best friend? What would they say? What weaknesses would they condemn? What strengths would they praise? Invite the client to write those down, and then to share a view of herself framed from this broader perspective.

Next the client can explore what roadblocks stand in the way of accepting herself as she is? Where would those roadblocks go on her matrix? Where would self-criticism and self-acceptance go, as toward moves or away moves (see Chapter 9)?

Another powerful way to validate clients and foster self-acceptance is to share some of your own struggles and imperfections. The goal here is not to put yourself center-stage nor to engage in one-upmanship, but simply to let the client see that you share in the common humanity of imperfection.

Working with Self-talk

You can help clients become more aware of their self-talk by inviting them to identify, in addition to what they think and feel in high-risk activity, how they talk to themselves, and what self-beliefs come with the self-talk.

In particular, do they experience thoughts and feelings of:

Feelings	Yes / No
Constant failure	❏ ❏
Worthlessness	❏ ❏
Imperfection	❏ ❏
Hopelessness	❏ ❏
Lack of control	❏ ❏
Dissatisfaction	❏ ❏
Insecurity	❏ ❏
Displeasure with themselves	❏ ❏
Depression	❏ ❏

Often self-talk is an act that clients deliberately engage in. It not only tells us about the content of their thoughts but evidences and constructs their positioning toward the world and their idiosyncratic worldview. This in turn affects the client's mood and behavior. Self-talk can become a hook that pulls clients into unworkable action and keeps them prisoners of the tic or habit loop, further feeding despair and self-loathing. However, for many clients, it can also be controlled to an extent. Invite your client to practice kinder and more validating self-talk and notice its effect on her and her behavior. Be sure to point out that you are not suggesting she should replace negative self-talk with positive affirmation, but rather she should validate her difficulties, give herself support and encouragement, expect and forgive missteps and setbacks, notice veering into unhelpful criticism, and consider that all humans stumble, fall, and fail at times.

When people with habits describe their inner states and their activities, they frequently report feelings of shame about themselves and low self-worth, guilt, and lack of control due to severe personal standards and unrealistic ideals of how they should act. Shame can also be internal and external, and is experienced as a vicious circle wherein shame about self, about perception of being judged and not living up to standards may trigger the habit.

This shame is also reflected in low mood and is maintained in the words and language the person uses to talk about herself and her problem. By having a more compassionate and self-compassionate stance as described above, the client can be encouraged to notice shaming self-talk and gradually develop kinder ways of speaking to herself (see self-compassionate and self-kindness exercises listed in Table 10.4 and Table 10.5). This in turn will positively impact her mood and how she perceives both her progress and inevitable setbacks. In this way, she will become less of a prisoner of her own thoughts and language. All humans are affected by the weight of symbolic functions of language and can often be at the mercy of the reactions they invoke. By becoming aware of how certain words trigger moods, tension, and critical or shaming self-talk, clients can learn more workable ways to conduct their inner dialogue. This powerful symbolic function of language is discussed in the next section.

Relational Frame Theory

Relational frame theory (RFT, Hayes, Roche,& Barnes-Holmes, 1999; Törneke, 2010), which underlies acceptance and commitment therapy (ACT), offers an account of the functioning of language processes that can throw light on how language, thoughts, emotions, and actions could play a role in the development and maintenance of tics and other habit disorders. RFT provides accounts for how symbolic stimuli, such as words, thoughts, and mental images can acquire physical and behavioral functions through a process known as the transformation of stimulus function. In Pavlov's famous experiments, pairing a bell sound with food delivery results in the bell sound acquiring the salivating physiological functions of the food, provided the neutral stimulus (the bell sound) is presented before the unconditioned stimulus of the food. Hayes and colleagues have shown that, in humans, language allows for a transformation of stimulus

Table 10.4 Kinder self-talk and metaphors

These are instructions we suggest you give to the client to encourage self-kindness and kinder self-talk.

Being kind to yourself

The following are tips on being kind to yourself:

Pay yourself compliments at least once per day on some aspect of your activities or appearance. This is not egotistical but just common recognition of who you are. The compliments can be fairly everyday and include comments about opening the door for someone; achieving a task like shopping; or helping a friend. Accept compliments from others with a simple: "That's kind of you." Or "Thank you very much." And pay compliments to others where appropriate, since this generates kind feelings in you

Remind yourself of your strengths and your positive aspects. That you can't always do what you wish but that your intentions and heart are in the right place

Be careful when you compare yourself with other people, since often we do this on only one dimension and we are multidimensional and have lots of dimensions that others do not

Remember to follow your reward schedule and regularly reward yourself each day, week, and month according to an unconditional schedule

Metaphors and analogies

Avoid negative metaphors when you describe difficulties that leave you passive and overwhelmed. Such as:

I'm trapped

I'm in a hole

I'm a broken machine

There is no light at the end of the tunnel

I'm the dummy in the class

I'm the person for whom nothing works

I'm on a slippery slope

I've a black cloud over me

Instead use positive metaphors or stories that place you actively and empowered in front of your difficulties:

I'm in some mud and brambles but I'll break free and carry on my hike

I've fallen into a ditch but I'll get out and carry on my way

I've slipped up temporarily on some ice but I'm okay to carry on

The light's ahead but I just need to get up closer

It's like learning to ride a bike: I'm going to fall off as part of learning the skill

Like everybody else I make my own mistakes but I own them and learn from them, which make me an intelligent learner

I'm skiing uphill and downhill but I'm in control and will arrive at the finish line

My weather is variable but it's mostly sunny days

functions, regardless of whether the neutral stimulus is presented before or after the unconditioned stimulus. They have further shown that this process also applies to symbolic or mental stimuli, meaning that by putting initially neutral stimuli such as words in relations with one another, their functions will transform. If the animal dog elicits fear and a readiness to flee, once put in relation with the animal, the sound "dog" can come to elicit fear and the premotor activation associated with a flight response. If the sound "dog" is put in an equivalent relation with the sound "perro," even in the absence of a dog, the Spanish word "perro" might come to acquire similar fear and premotor functions

Table 10.5 Self-compassionate exercises

Below are suggested guidelines to encourage self-compassion in the client.

1) Accept critical voices. Accepting and validating them does not make them real. They are just thoughts, and acknowledging them does not mean you should act on them

2) Answer the voice gently but assertively by asserting your trust in yourself and your decisions; recapitulate your strong points; understand your performance in the context of its occurrence and the circumstances and not in a judgment after the fact

3) You have many talents and many successes that testify to your worth. In any case living is a question of learning and nobody's life is without ups and downs. It is a question of what you take away from your learning experiences

4) Often feelings of frustration, dissatisfaction, and failure are natural reactions to the way you set yourself up to fail. We saw this concretely with your adoption of styles of action that seemed valid but in fact created unnecessary tension and were self-sabotaging

5) Use the mindfulness exercises of detachment to observe the critical thoughts. Who or where do they arise from? Where do they get their authority to talk like this to you? Do they come from an identifiable person or authority in the past?

6) Take a stand in replying to them. Accept them and their point of view but reply with a more compassionate voice to counterbalance their negativity
e.g., "I am not worthless and useless because of one event or feeling, I have many strengths including the strength to learn, I cope well with many difficult circumstances so your judgment is not appropriate or accurate reflection of me and my strengths."
It is particularly important to realize that a negative critical voice is:
Depressing; demoralizing; unconstructive (it goes nowhere and is paralyzing); it is too narrow and rigid a reflection of who you are; it is essentially an opinion or an unjustified statement. Comparatively, a constructive compassionate voice is: respectful and centered on you and your welfare; is realistic in drawing on your strengths; leads to further options; and is encouraging of your worth and ability to effect further action.

---

to the animal. This process soon leads to an explosion of relations and the establishment of complex relational networks in which the transformation of function is controlled by contextual cues that specify the relations such as "bigger than" or "worse than." As different stimuli are related (or framed) through these contextual cues, functions are transformed—a process known as derived relational responding. For example, if the client is afraid of big dogs and the client hears that a German shepherd dog is one of the biggest dogs, the fear activation functions of other dogs will now transfer, augmented, to German shepherd dogs, even if the client never has never met one. The client's reaction to the thought of a German shepherd dog is a derived relational response, and it will likely involve premotor activation somewhat similar to being in the presence of the animal. This process is largely involuntary and could also influence the links between thought, emotion, and action that underlie tic and habits disorders, as the premotor activation linked to the appearance of aversive or appetitive stimuli in the world of physical experience can now attach to thoughts or anticipations, through the derived functions they can acquire. Thus, a person with tics or habits might fear being judged as they perform an action. The thought of being judged comes with tension as a derived function, so the person will tense up the instant the thought shows up. Similarly, a person with perfectionistic standards will approach tasks with assumptions that include derived functions leading to muscular tension. RFT suggests novel ways of targeting these functions rather than trying to change the networks themselves.

An RFT-inspired Link between Dysfunctional Thoughts and Tension

RFT alerts us to the largely automatic buildup of relational networks. It also suggests that trying to intervene with the members of the networks by trying to replace them may in fact increase the activation of these members. The simplest example of that is trying to replace one thought by another, as in the pink unicorn example given in Chapter 9. Seemingly sophisticated strategies for replacing one thought with another by seeking evidence for the thought may run into the same problems. They may produce more "evidence" for the dysfunctional thought as the network activates around the targeted cognition, rather than lead to its replacement. For a client fearing others will judge his tic or habit, the observable absence of evidence of people loudly judging him may generate more reasons as to why people would not dare to share their judgments, maybe precisely because they are highly negative. The risk is thus further entanglement with the thought.

For this reason, RFT suggests a more effective strategy might be to notice the thought, and notice its functions. For people with tics, the function of a thought about being judged or an assumption about having to be perfect, will be an increase in muscular tension. When that function is noticed, the client can practice releasing tension. The noticing hooks and what you do next metaphor, with special emphasis on muscle tension, can get clients to effectively decouple problematic thoughts and assumptions from their function in creating or maintaining tension.

For this work you can use a special adaptation of the hooks worksheet for tic and habit disorders. In addition to the thought, emotion, or anticipation that can hook clients and that they can write on the bait, there is a space to write which muscles they tense up (the fishing line) and what action it leads them too (the box at the end of the line) (see Figure 9.3).

For clinicians and clients, a potential advantage of this approach is not getting entangled in arguments about the rationality or realistic nature of particular thoughts or assumptions. Further, as clients come to loosen up some of the behavioral functions of thoughts and assumptions, they gradually come to take them less seriously and feel less of an urge to act on them. Here too using the matrix to help clients sort thoughts, emotions, and the behavior (whether moves away or moves toward) that follows them, can help.

Therapist checklist for dealing with emotions

Client identifies emotions linked to the tic or habit	Yes / No ❏ ❏
The client can fill in the habit–shame loop.	Yes / No ❏ ❏
The client identifies self-focused criticism with examples	Yes / No ❏ ❏
The client accepts self and emotions uncritically and is self-compassionate over frustrations	Yes / No ❏ ❏
The client notices hooks on words and expressions, and how they may react and tense up to certain habitual phrases	Yes / No ❏ ❏
The client is able to move beyond the association and move on	Yes / No ❏ ❏

11

Achieving Goals and Maintaining Gains

Maintaining the New Behavior

The new habit of preventing tension buildup, particularly since it involves doing less and more economically, can be installed in a matter of a few weeks, but we advise the client to keep actively practicing strategies for mastering tension for up to 3 months, and with continued practice there is continued improvement (please fill in Table 11.1). It is particularly important to be especially vigilant during periods of high stress, since there is a tendency to revert back to earlier patterns of behavior at that time. Also when new situations arise that are similar to old high risk ones, it is important to apply the strategies the client has found useful. Much of the program already completed will apply to any new tic or habit, and the client will already have gained insight into his or her problem. We have supplied tables to help plan ahead for future problems (see Table 11.1).

New tics or habits

If the client has several tic or habit problems, deal with each one in order of priority or begin with the least complicated problem and progress to the most difficult. Because the emphasis of our program is on processes building up to tics and habits, there is usually a general effect of the treatment on other tics.

We advise that the client should master one tic or habit before progressing to another. Moreover, knowledge gained from past tics or habits and tension regarding relaxation and mindfulness, styles of action, planning less, and linking thoughts and action should apply to all subsequent tics or habits.

The application of the program to another tic or habit follows the same principles as the first application, and should be smoother given prior experience and expectation.

Do not move on to another habit until the client reports mastery of the first habit. If there is a greater than 90% improvement in one of the parameters (frequency, intensity, control), as determined by self-report of the client's control of his or her problem in the targeted activity, then go onto the next activity, but continue practicing mastery of the first tic or habit.

Managing Tic and Habit Disorders: A Cognitive Psychophysiological Approach with Acceptance Strategies, First Edition. Kieron P O'Connor, Marc E Lavoie, and Benjamin Schoendorff.
© 2017 John Wiley & Sons, Ltd. Published 2017 by John Wiley & Sons, Ltd.
Companion Website: www.wiley.com/go/oconnor/managingticandhabitdsorders

Table 11.1 Follow-up questionnaire

1. Were improvements accomplished during the therapy program maintained?

									During the past week		
a) Frequency	Number of units[a]										
b) Control	0	10	20	30	40	50	60	70	80	90	100
c) Intensity	0	10	20	30	40	50	60	70	80	90	100
d) General level of tension	0	10	20	30	40	50	60	70	80	90	100
	(tense)								(relaxed)		

2. (a) If the improvement weren't maintained, for what reason(s)?

_____

_____

2. (b) What could be done to improve adhesion to the treatment? (Discuss this with the client)

_____

_____

3. (a) Which exercises does the client use regularly? Specify.

_____

_____

3. (b) Are they useful?

_____

_____

4. (a) Were the exercises generalized to another tic or another habit? If yes, specify.

_____

_____

4. (b) Does the generalization work?

_____

_____

5. Were there any major changes in:

(a) The clients life?

_____

_____

(b) The behavior of the client?

_____

_____

(c) The emotional state of the client?

_____

_____

(d) The physical form of the client?

_____

_____

(e) Medication or other interventions?

_____

_____

(continued)

6. Did the changes in the tic or habit of the client result in other impacts on his or her quality of life? Specify.

_____

_____

7. To what degree is the client confident he/she will continue to improve in the control of his/her tics or habits (0–100%)? In the control of his/her levels of tension (0–100%)?

_____

_____

8. (a) What does the client consider to be the difficulties related to continuing or making progress in using the key strategies of the program (attention, relaxation, discrimination, style of action, appropriate response, cognitive restructuration, relapse prevention)? (Cover each of the strategies and note the response)

_____

_____

_____

8. (b) Does the client believe he/she needs more information or coaching? If yes, specify.

_____

_____

_____

8. (c) Did you do coaching during the interview? If yes, specify.

_____

_____

9. Have other individuals made positive or negative comments about the client's progress? Specify.

_____

_____

10. Were there any other comments from the client on his/her progress or on the program?

_____

_____

_____

Note: [a] Check that the units are the same as those in the notebook.

The protocol to follow in dealing with the tic or habit:

1) Target the new tic or habit and describe it and monitor it with the video and daily diary and a close other.
2) Examine variation and detail the high and low risk activities triggering the tic or habit.
3) Elicit evaluations and trace thoughts and feelings specific to the tic or habit.
4) Link to styles of action to anticipations and assumptions and background beliefs.
5) Ensure the client completes the exercises for improving cognitive and physical flexibility with this tic or habit.
6) Practice exercises relevant to the tic or habit evaluation.
7) Continue to fill in the self-confidence rating.
8) Get feedback from the diary.

Feedback

Feedback on the new performance is especially important to maintaining the new habit since it rewards the person for changing the habit and monitoring progress straight away indicates progress.

The first type of feedback is self-feedback, where the client asks him/herself each day:

1) Is the problem worse or better? By how much?
2) To what degree has control improved?
3) How confident is the client about gaining more control?
4) Does the client feel more relaxed and comfortable overall?

Apart from the objective observations of the frequency of the problem, the client can also note whether his/her degree of confidence about changing other aspects of his or her life has increased and whether this has led to more successful outcomes in personal affairs and relationships. Has success in control and mastery of the movement problem led to change in other habits or aspects of life?

Another source of feedback is the comments of others: family, friends, B.e.s.t. Buddy and associates. Often people will give their encouraging remarks unsolicited but, if not, try to get the client to seek feedback from them and their comments on how the client's appearance has changed. The client can seek feedback from acquaintances they trust on his or her new habit. Encouraging sympathetic remarks from close and trusted others provide good positive feedback.

Sensory feedback is also important. This involves getting direct physiological feedback from a new posture or movement about its new state. The client can be encouraged to check the newer relaxed state mentally or manually and feel the benefit of relief. All types of feedback are important in changing and maintaining thinking and muscle patterns.

The final feedback is planning regular rewards for the efforts in doing less effort and in changing tension level. Plan with the client a regular reward schedule for: every day, every week and every month, in accordance with practice and progress.

New Situations

It is particularly important to be vigilant in applying the strategies during stressful moments, or when the client is tired, or when he or she is on holiday, or when faced with an entirely new situation. It may be worth sitting down now and reflecting on what new situations might be likely to resemble high risk situations in order to be better prepared.

The procedure to follow here is: (a) identify the new tic or habit; (b) look at its situational profile; (c) look at evaluation and thoughts associated with the tic; (d) identify the style of action associated with the new tic; (e) practice discrimination, relaxation, and thought and muscle flexibility as appropriate; and finally (f) practice the new strategy (see Table 11.2).

Table 11.2 Planning for possible triggers for relapse

List below any new or repeat contexts of activities that you consider at risk to trigger the urge to tic.

New context/activity	Tic elicited	Solution
Example:		
Holiday in Spain	Eye blink	Practice relaxation and be flexible with personal style of action and associated thoughts

Reward and Self-compassion

The client should seek regular rewards for his or her efforts and remember to highlight accomplishments—the tics or habits reduced, not just those still remaining. Remember the glass can be half-full or half-empty in terms of the client's progress, but which version the client chooses can affect mood and optimism. A very important part of the program is accepting the tic or habit and being non-judgmental. Part of being flexible and letting go is not thinking rigidly, as we identified in the thoughts leading to tension and emotions: accepting emotions and sensations and trying to cope with them positively.

The other core notion in relapse prevention is that the client should define him or herself as a person apart from the tics or habits. Go back to the goal and inconveniences we specified and look back at what the client feels free to do. Now is the time to adopt other behaviors that define the client as a non-tic person. Such new habits will reinforce the client's new non-tic habits and identity. Fix a schedule to deal with the remaining tics.

The client can justifiably define him or herself more and more as someone who does not tic or habit and is not a tic or habit sufferer since most of his or her life does not feature ticking.

Relapse Prevention

The types of event likely to lead to relapse are: fatigue, positive and negative stress, depression or just feeling sad, being too occupied, illness, major environment or life changes, traumatizing events, alcohol, drugs, interpersonal conflict, and all feelings of insecurity.

Other factors that may precipitate a temporary relapse are: not all the tics or habits have been addressed, the strategies have not been continuously applied, there is difficulty with one or more components of the program, there is an absence of positive support, there is a difficulty in eliminating tension, or there is a difficulty in generating new strategies for other tics or habits. The tic or habit may well come back temporarily, but if it does, it is important not to feel that the tic or habit has returned for good. It is merely a slip from which the person can recover. All relapses can be viewed as *temporary*, not as final and a catastrophe; refer to the manual at the appropriate place if the client feels unsure of a strategy. The key to relapse prevention is to continue to put the exercises into practice, as the program draws on strengths and eventually encourages the client to feel more accepting and compassionate towards him or herself. The new non-tic habit should be integrated quickly into the client's routine. The risk of relapse seems to be lower if the person has changed his or her style of planning, and puts time into carrying out the practice exercises, or has changed his or her lifestyle.

The client knows enough now about triggers for his or her tics or habits and tension, and so on. He or she should be able to trace the activity or environmental signal that triggered the tic or habit and adapt for next time, learning how to deal with new high risk situations to avoid relapse in the future. If the client has a bad day he or she may find him/herself momentarily relapsing into a bad way of acting, just like tumbling off a bike. Ask the client the following questions: What was the reason for the relapse? What strategies did I not employ? How can this knowledge help me prevent relapse in the future (see Table 11.3)?

The client can continue to receive feedback regularly on progress—even if he or she has no tics or habits. External support continues to be important throughout recovery.

If other tics or habits occur, apply the program to these tics or habits.

The client can always keep in mind the main components of the program that were helpful, deal with new high risk situations on the basis of knowledge, and plan a calendar of new reinforcements for continuing practice of the program. This calendar can be integrated into a new lifestyle and the client should continue to receive social support and encouragement from his or her B.e.s.t. Buddy.

Achieving Non-tic Goals

It may now also be a good idea for the client to change other aspects of his or her life for the better: maybe quit smoking, take up exercise as a new hobby, or start a new course. It is important for the client to receive positive feedback for his or her newfound tension-free life and non-tic self, perhaps by exposure to social situations that previously he or she may have avoided. Increase in confidence helps avoid relapse.

Table 11.3 Components of the therapy you found useful

Components of the therapy	Helpfulness rating
Education on tics	_____
Awareness training	_____
Video	_____
Daily diary	_____
Style of action	_____
Flexibility, becoming more flexible	_____
Relaxation	_____
Tolerating the sensation	_____
Mindfulness and self-compassion	_____
The ACT Matrix	_____
Self-talk	_____
Metaphors	_____
Social support and B.e.s.t. Buddy support	_____
Boosting confidence	_____

Dimension								
1	2	3	4	5	6	7	8	9
Not helpful at all		A little helpful	Somewhat helpful		Very helpful		Extremely helpful	

Clients have reported the following gains in other spheres of life: the *majority* of our clients reported the following strategies as helpful—style of action, tension management, and external support from the therapist and other people. Thoughts about tic or habit onset changed naturally as a consequence of the program and clients were generally less distressed.

Participants were better able to prioritize activities, complete tasks more satisfactorily, showed an improvement in mood (e.g., frustration), found themselves less in conflict situations, were better at delegating to others, had a realistic appreciation of the self and self-accomplishments, and a better grasp of plans of action and what can be realistically accomplished. Knowledge is power, and if the client has completed all stages of the program it is very unlikely that he or she will return to pre-treatment program levels of ticking. The client would have to work hard to unlearn and unpractice the program.

Finally

1) Stay aware of tension level at all times as well as his or her anticipations, particularly in difficult situations.
2) Be conscious of the continual coupling of thought, mood, and action.

3) Continue regular application of strategies.
4) Be flexible in approach to tic and habit related thoughts and action, particularly a habitual action.
5) In case of a slip identify the section of the manual relevant to the type of slip and re-read it.
6) If he or she has a bad day, he/she should not despair; consider what strategies he/she needs to revise.
7) Adopt new activities to reinforce his or her non-tic status.

Bravo! The therapist can award the client with the certificate of accomplishment.

References

Anderson, M. T., Vu, C., Derby, K. M., Goris, M., & McLaughlin, T. F. (2002). Using functional analysis procedures to monitor medication effects in an outpatient and school setting. *Psychology in the Schools, 39*(11), 73–76.

APA (American Psychiatric Association) (2000). *Diagnostic and statistical manual of mental disorders* (4th edition). Washington DC: American Psychiatric Association.

APA (American Psychiatric Association) (2013). *Diagnostic and statistical manual of mental disorders* (5th edition). Washington DC: Elsevier.

Ascher, E. (1948). Psychodynamic considerations in Gilles de la Tourette's disease, maladie des tics, with a report of 5 cases and discussion of the literature. *American Journal of Psychiatry, 105*(4), 267–276.

Azrin, N. H., & Nunn, R. G. (1973). Habit-reversal: A method of eliminating nervous habits and tics. *Behavior Research and Therapy, 11*(4), 619–628.

Azrin, N. H., & Nunn, R .G. (1977). *Habit control in a day*. New York: Simon & Schuster.

Bloch, M. H., Landeros-Weisenberger, A., Dombrowski, P., Kelmendi, B., Wegner, R., Nudel, J., & Coric, V. (2007). Systematic review: Pharmacological and behavioral treatment for trichotillomania. *Biological Psychiatry, 62*(8), 839–846. doi:10.1016/j.biopsych.2007.05.019

Bohlhalter, S., Goldfine, A., Matteson, S., Garraux, G., Hanakawa, T., Kansaku, K., & Hallett, M. (2006). Neural correlates of tic generation in Tourette syndrome: An event-related functional MRI study. *Brain, 129*(8), 2029–2037. doi:10.1093/brain/awl050

Bond, F. W., Hayes, S. C., Baer, R. A., Carpenter, K. M., Guenole, N., Orcutt, H. K., Waltz, T., & Zettle, R. D. (2011). Preliminary psychometric properties of the Acceptance and Action Questionnaire—II: A revised measure of psychological inflexibility and experiential avoidance. *Behavior Therapy, 42*(4): 676–888.

Branet, I., Hosatte-Ducassy, C., O'Connor, K. P., & Lavoie, M. E. (2010). Motor processing and brain activity are related to cognitive-behavioral improvement in chronic tic and habit disorders. *International Journal of Psychophysiology, 77*(3).

Catrou, J. (1890). Étude sur la maladie des tics convulsifs. Thèse pour le doctorat en médecine. No 129. Bibliothèque interuniversitaire de médecine (Paris, Jouve). Retrieved from www.bium.univ-paris5.fr/histmed/medica/cote?TPAR1890x129

Managing Tic and Habit Disorders: A Cognitive Psychophysiological Approach with Acceptance Strategies, First Edition. Kieron P O'Connor, Marc E Lavoie, and Benjamin Schoendorff.
© 2017 John Wiley & Sons, Ltd. Published 2017 by John Wiley & Sons, Ltd.
Companion Website: www.wiley.com/go/oconnor/managingticandhabitdsorders

Cavanna, A. E., David, K., Bandera, V., Termine, C., Balottin, U., Schrag, A., & Selai, C. (2013). Health-related quality of life in Gilles de la Tourette syndrome: A decade of research. *Behavioural Neurology, 27*(1), 83–93. doi:10.3233/ben-120296

Cavanna, A. E., David, K., Orth, M., & Robertson, M. M. (2012). Predictors during childhood of future health-related quality of life in adults with Gilles de la Tourette syndrome. *European Journal of Paediatric Neurology, 16*(6), 605–612.

Christenson, G. A., & Crow, S. J. (1996). The characterization and treatment of trichotillomania. *Journal of Clinical Psychiatry, 57*, 42–47.

Corbett, J. A., Mathews, A. M., Connell, P. H., & Shapiro, D. A. (1969). Tics and Gilles de la Tourette's syndrome: A follow-up study and critical review. *British Journal of Psychiatry, 115*(528), 1229–1241.

Crossley, E., & Eugenio Cavanna, A. (2013). Sensory phenomena: Clinical correlates and impact on quality of life in adult patients with Tourette syndrome. *Psychiatry Research, 209*(3), 709–710. doi: https://dx.doi.org/10.1016/j.psychres.2013.04.019

Dana, C. L., & Wilkin, W. P. (1886). On convulsive tic with explosive disturbances of speech (so-called Gilles de la Tourette's disease). *Journal of Nervous and Mental Disease, 13*(7), 407–412.

Devilly, G. J., & Borkovec, T. D. (2000). Psychometric properties of the Credibility/ Expectancy Questionnaire. *Journal of Behavior Therapy and Experimental Psychiatry, 31*(2), 73–86. doi:10.1016/S0005-7916(00)00012-4

Deckersbach, T., Chou, T., Britton, J. C., Carlson, L. E., Reese, H. E., Siev, J., & Wilhelm, S. (2014). Neural correlates of behavior therapy for Tourette's disorder. *Psychiatry Research, 224*(3), 269–274. doi:10.1016/j.pscychresns.2014.09.003

Falkenstein, M. J., Mouton-Odum, S., Mansueto, C. S., Golomb, R. G., &. Haaga, D. A. F. (2015). Comprehensive behavioral treatment of trichotillomania: A treatment development study. *Behavior Modification, 40*(3), 414–438. doi:10.1177/0145445515616369

Ferenczi, S. (1921). Psycho-analytical observation on tic. *International Journal of Psycho-Analysis*, 1–30.

Fine, K. M., Walther, M. R., Joseph, J. M., Robinson, J., Ricketts, E. J., Bowe, W. E., & Woods, D. W. (2012). Acceptance-enhanced behavior therapy for trichotillomania in adolescents. *Cognitive Behavioral Practice, 19*, 463–471.

Flessner, C. A., Busch, A. M., Heideman, P. W., & Woods, D. W. (2008a). Acceptance-Enhanced Behavior Therapy (AEBT) for trichotillomania and chronic skin picking: Exploring the effects of component sequencing. *Behavior Modification, 32*(5), 579–594.

Flessner, C. A., Conelea, C. A., Woods, D. W., Franklin, M. E., Keuthen, N. J., & Cashin, S. E. (2008b). Style of pulling in trichotillomania: Exploring differences in symptom severity, phenomenology, and functional impact. *Behaviour Research and Therapy, 46*, 345–357.

Flessner, C. A., Woods, D. W., Franklin, M. E., Cashin, S. E., Keuthen, N. J., & Board, T. L. C. S. A. (2008c). The Milwaukee inventory for subtype of trichotillomania-adult version (MIST-A): development of an instrument for the assessment of "focused" and "automatic" hair pulling. *Journal of Psychopathology and Behavioral Assessment, 30*(1), 20–30.

Freeman, R. D. (2007). Tourette Syndrome International Database Consortium. Tic disorders and ADHD: answers from a world-wide clinical dataset on Tourette syndrome. *European and Child Adolescent Psychiatry, 16*(Suppl 1), 15–23.

Freeman, R. D., Fast, D. K., Burd, L., Kerbeshian, J., Robertson, M. M., & Sandor, P. (2000). An international perspective on Tourette syndrome: Selected findings from 3,500 individuals in 22 countries. *Developmental Medicine and Child Neurology, 42*(7), 436–447.

Gelinas, B. L., & Gagnon, M. M. (2013). Pharmacological and psychological treatments of pathological skin-picking: A preliminary meta-analysis .*Journal of Obsessive Compulsive Related Disorders, 2*(2), 167–175. doi:https://dx.doi.org/10.1016/j.jocrd.2013.02.003

George, M.S.,Trimble, M.R., Ring, H.A., Sallee, F.R., & Robertson, M.M. (1993). Obsessions in Obsessive-Compulsive disorder with and without Gilles de la Tourette's syndrome. *American Journal of Psychiatry, 150*(1), 93–97.

Gillanders, D. T., Bolderston, H., Bond, F. W., Dempster, M., Flaxman, P. E., Campbell, L., . . . & Remington, B. (2014). The development and initial validation of the Cognitive Fusion Questionnaire. *Behavior Therapy, 45*, 83–101.

Gilles de la Tourette, G. (1885). Étude sur une affection nerveuse caractérisée par de l'incoordination motrice accompagnée d'écholalie et de coprolalie. *Archives de Neurologie, 9*, 19–42, 158–200.

Golden, G. S. (1974). Gilles de la Tourette's syndrome following methylphenidate administration. *Developmental Medicine and Child Neurology, 16*, 76–78.

Gratz, K. L., & Roemer, L. (2004). Multidimensional assessment of emotion regulation and dysregulation: Development, factor structure, and initial validation of the difficulties in emotion regulation scale. *Journal of Psychopathology and Behavioral Assessment, 26*(1), 41–54.

Harcherik, D. F., Leckman, J. F., Detlor, J., & Cohen, D. J. (1984). A new instrument for clinical studies of Tourette's syndrome. *Journal of the American Academy for Child Psychiatry, 23*(2), 153–160.

Hayes, S. C., Barnes-Holmes, D., & Roche, B. (Eds.). (2001). *Relational Frame Theory: A post-Skinnerian account of human language and cognition.* New York: Plenum Press.

Hayes, S. C, Strosahl, K. D., & Wilson, K. G. (2012). *Acceptance and commitment therapy: The process and practice of mindful change* (2nd edition). New York: The Guilford Press.

Hornsey, H., Banerjee, S., Zeitlin, H., & Robertson, M. (2001). The prevalence of Tourette syndrome in 13–14-year-olds in mainstream schools. *Journal of Child Psychology and Psychiatry, 42*(8), 1035–1039.

Itard, J.-M. G. (1825). Mémoire sur quelques fonctions involontaires des appareils de la locomotion, de la préhension et de la voix. *Archives Générales de Médecine, Série 1*(8), 385–406. Retrieved from www.biusante.parisdescartes.fr/histoire/medica/resultats/?p=385&cote=90165x1825x08&do=page

Kadesjö, B., & Gillberg, C. J. (2000). Tourette's disorder: Epidemiology and comorbidity in primary school children. *American Academy of Child and Adolescent Psychiatry, 39*(5), 548–555.

Kataria, M. (2012). *The inner spirit of laughter: Five secrets from the laughing guru.* India: Dr Kataria School of Laughter Yoga.

Keuthen, N. J., Flessner, C. A., Woods, D. W., Franklin, M. E., Stein, D. J., & Cashin, S. E. (2007). Factor analysis of the Massachusetts General Hospital Hairpulling Scale. *Journal of Psychosomatic Research, 62*(2), 707–709.

Keuthen, N. J., O'Sullivan, R. L., Ricciardi, J. N., Shera, D., Savage, C. R., Borgmann, A. S., Jenike, M. A., & Baaer, L. (1995). The Massachusetts General Hospital (MGH) Hairpulling Scale: 1. Development and Factor Analyses. *Psychotherapy and Psychosomatics, 64*, 141–145.

Keuthen, N. J., Rothbaum, B. O., Fama, J., Altenberger, E., Falkenstein, M. J., Sprich, S. E., Kearns, M., Meunier, S., Jenicke, M. A., & Welch, S. S. (2012). DBT-enhanced cognitive-behavioral treatment for trichotillomania: A randomized controlled trial. *Journal of Behavioral Addiction, 1*(3), 106–114.

Keuthen, N. J., Tung, E. S., Woods, D. W., Franklin, M. E., Altenburger, E. M., Pauls, D. L., & Flessner, C. A. (2015). Replication study of the Milwaukee Inventory for Subtypes of Trichotillomania—Adult Version in a clinically characterized sample. *Behavior Modification, 39*(4), 590–599.

Keuthen, N. J., Wilhelm, S., Deckersbach, T., Engelhard, I. M., Forker, A.E., Baer, L., & Jenike, M. A. (2001). The Skin Picking Scale: Scale construction and psychometric analyses. *Journal of Psychosomatic Research, 50*(6), 337–341.

Kramer, H., & Sprenger, J. (1948). *Malleus maleficarum.* Translated by Reverend Montague Summers. London: Pushkin Press.

Lanzi, G., Zambrino, C. A., Termine, C., Palestra, M., Ferrari Ginevra, O., Orcesi, S., Manfredi, P., & Beghi, E., (2004). Prevalence of tic disorders among primary school students in the city of Pavia, Italy. *Archives of the Diseased Child, 89*(1), 45–47.

Lavoie, M. E., Imbriglio, T. V., Stip, E., & O'Connor, K. P. (2011). Neurocognitive changes following cognitive-behavioral treatment in the Tourette syndrome and chronic tic disorder. *International Journal of Cognitive Psychotherapy, 4*(2), 34–50.

Lavoie, M. E., Leclerc, J., & O'Connor, K. P. (2013). Bridging neuroscience and clinical psychology: Cognitive behavioral and psychophysiological models in the evaluation and treatment of Gilles de la Tourette syndrome. *Neuropsychiatry (London), 3*(1), 75–87. doi:10.2217/npy.12.70

Leckman, J. F., Riddle M. A., Hardin, M. T., Orth, S. I., Swartz, K.L., Stevenson, J., & Cohen, D, J. (1989). The Yale Global Tic Severity Scale: Initial testing of a clinician-rated scale of tic severity. *Journal of the American Academy of Child and Adolescent Psychiatry, 28*(4), 566–573.

Leclerc, J., Forget, J., & O'Connor, K. P. (Eds) (2008) *Quand le corps fait à sa tête. Le syndrome Gilles de la Tourette.* Québec: Éditions Multimondes.

Lombroso, P. J., Scahill, L., King, R. A., Lynch, K. A., Chappell, P. B., Peterson, B. S., McDougle, C. J., & Leckman, J. F. (1995). Risperidone treatment of children and adolescents with chronic tic disorders: A preliminary report. *Journal of the American Academy of Child and Adolescent Psychiatry, 34*(9), 1147–1152.

Mahler, M. S. (1944). Tics and impulsions in children: A study of motility. *The Psychoanalytic Quarterly, xiii*, 430–444.

Mahler, M. S., Luke, J. A., & Daltroff, W. (1945). Clinical and follow-up study of the tic syndrome in children. *American Journal of Orthopsychiatry, xv*, 631–647.

Mansueto, C. S., Golomb, R. G., Thomas, A. M., & Stemberger, R. M. T. (1999). A comprehensive model for behavioral treatment of trichotillomania. *Cognitive and Behavioral Practice, 99*, 23–43.

Marcks, B. A., Berlin, K. S., Woods, D. W., & Davies, W. H. (2007). Impact of Tourette syndrome: A preliminary investigation of the effects of disclosure on peer perceptions and social functioning. *Psychiatry, 70*(1), 59–67.

Mason, A., Banerjee, S., Eapen, V., Zeitlin, H., Robertson, M. M. (1998). The prevalence of Tourette syndrome in a mainstream school population. *Developmental Medicine and Child Neurology, 40*(5), 292–296.

McGuire, J. F., Piacentini, J., Brennan, E. A., Lewin, A. B., Murphy, T. K., Small, B. J., & Storch, E. A. (2014). A meta-analysis of behavior therapy for Tourette Syndrome. *Journal of Psychiatric Research, 50*, 106–112. doi:10.1016/j. jpsychires.2013.12.009

McGuire, J. F., Ung, D., Selles, R. R., Rahman, O., Lewin, A. B., Murphy, T. K., & Storch, E. A. (2014). Treating trichotillomania: A meta-analysis of treatment effects and moderators for behavior therapy and serotonin reuptake inhibitors. *Journal of Psychiatric Research, 58*, 76–83. doi:10.1016/j.jpsychires.2014.07.015

Morand-Beaulieu, S., O'Connor, K. P., Richard, M., Sauve, G., Leclerc, J. B., Blanchet, P. J., & Lavoie, M. E. (2016). The impact of a cognitive-behavioral therapy on event-related potentials in patients with tic disorders or body-focused repetitive behaviors. *Frontiers in Psychiatry, 7*, 81. doi:10.3389/fpsyt.2016.00081

Morand-Beaulieu, S., O'Connor, K. P., Sauve, G., Blanchet, P. J., & Lavoie, M. E. (2015). Cognitive-behavioral therapy induces sensorimotor and specific electrocortical changes in chronic tic and Tourette's disorder. *Neuropsychologia, 79*(B), 310–321. doi:10.1016/j.neuropsychologia.2015.05.024

Muller-Vahl, K. R., Berding, G., Brucke, T., Kolbe, H., Meyer, G. J., Hundeshagen, H., & Emrich, H. M. (2000). Dopamine transporter binding in Gilles de la Tourette syndrome. *Journal of Neurology, 247*(7), 514–520.

Norberg, M. M., Wetterneck, C. T., Woods, D. W., & Conelea, C. A. (2007). Examination of the mediating role of psychological acceptance in relationships between cognitions and severity of chronic hairpulling. *Behavior Modification, 31*, 367–381.

O'Connor, K. P. (2001). Clinical and psychological features distinguishing obsessive-compulsive and chronic tic disorders. *Clinical Psychology Review, 20*(8), 1–30.

O'Connor, K. P. (2002). A cognitive behavioral/psychophysiological model of tic disorders. Invited Essay. *Behavior Research and Therapy, 40*, 1113–1142.

O'Connor, K. P. (2005). *Cognitive-behavioral management of tic disorders.* New York: John Wiley & Sons Ltd.

O'Connor, K. P., & Aardema, F. (Eds.). (2012). *Clinician's handbook for obsessive compulsive disorder.* Chichester: John Wiley & Sons Ltd.

O'Connor, K. P., Brault, M., Robillard, S., Loiselle, J., Borgeat, F., & Stip, E. (2001). Evaluation of a cognitive-behavioural program for the management of chronic tic and habit disorders. *Behavioral Research and Therapy, 39*(6), 667–681.

O'Connor, K. P., Laverdure, A., Taillon, A., Stip, E., Borgeat, F., & Lavoie, M. (2009). Cognitive behavioral management of Tourette's syndrome and chronic tic disorder in medicated and unmedicated samples. *Behaviour Research and Therapy, 47*(12), 1090–1095. doi:10.1016/j.brat.2009.07.021

O'Connor, K. P., Lavoie, M., Blanchet, P., & St-Pierre-Delorme, M. È. (2015). Evaluation of a cognitive psychophysiological model for management of tic disorders: an open trial. *The British Journal of Psychiatry*. doi:10.1192/bjp. bp.114.154518

O'Connor, K. P., Lavoie, M. E., Robert, M., Stip, E., & Borgeat, F. (2005). Brain-behavior relations during motor processing in chronic tic and habit disorder. *Cognitive and Behavioral Neurology, 18*(2), 79–88.

O'Connor, K. P., Lavoie, M. E., Stip, E., Borgeat, F., & Laverdure, A. (2008). Cognitive-behaviour therapy and skilled motor performance in adults with chronic tic disorder. *Neuropsychological Rehabilitation, 18*(1), 45–64. doi:10.1080/09602010701390835

O'Connor, K. P., St-Pierre Delorme, M.-E., Leclerc, J., Lavoie, M. T., & Blais, M. (2014). Meta-cognitions in Tourette syndrome, tic disorder, and body-focused repetitive disorder. *Canadian Journal of Psychiatry, 59*(8), 417–425.

Pélissier, M.-C., & O'Connor, K. P. (2004) Cognitive-behavioral treatment for trichotillomania, targeting perfectionism. *Clinical Case Studies, 3*(1), 57–69.

Penzel, F. (1995). Skin picking and nail biting: Related habits. *In Touch. 1*, 1–10.

Peterson, B. S. (2001). Neuroimaging studies of Tourette syndrome: A decade of progress. *Advances in Neurology, 85*, 179–196.

Peterson, B. S., Staib, L., Scahill, L., Zhang, H., Anderson, C., Leckman, J. F., & Webster, R. (2001). Regional brain and ventricular volumes in Tourette syndrome. *Archives of General Psychiatry, 58*(5), 427–440.

Peterson, B. S., Thomas, P., Kane, M. J., Scahill, L., Zhang, H., Bronen, R., & Staib, L. (2003). Basal ganglia volumes in patients with Gilles de la Tourette syndrome. *Archives of General Psychiatry, 60*(4), 415–424.

Pringsheim, T., Doja, A., Gorman, D., McKinlay, D., Day, L., Billinghurst, L., & Sandor, P. (2012). Canadian guidelines for the evidence-based treatment of tic disorders: Pharmacotherapy. *Canadian Journal of Psychiatry, 57*(3), 133–143.

Pringsheim, T., & Marras, C. (2009). Pimozide for tics in Tourette's syndrome. *Cochrane Database Systematic Reviews, 2*, CD006996. doi:10.1002/14651858. CD006996.pub2

Riddle, M. A., Leckman, J. F., Anderson, G. M., Hardin, M. T., Ort, S. I., Towbin, K. E., Shaywitz, B. A., & Cohen, D. J. (1987). Assessment of dopaminergic function in children and adults: Long and brief debrisoquin administration combined with plasma homovanillic acid. *Psychopharmacology Bulletin, 23*(3), 411–414.

Roane, H. S., Piazza, C. C., Cercone, J. J., & Grados, M. (2002). Assessment and treatment of vocal tics associated with Tourette's syndrome. *Behavior Modification, 26*(4), 482–498.

Roberts, S., O'Connor, K. P., Aardema, F., & Bélanger, C. (2015). The impact of emotions on body-focused repetitive behaviors: Evidence from a non-treatment-seeking sample. *Journal of Behavior Therapy and Experimental Psychiatry, 46*, 189–197.

Roberts, S., O'Connor, K. P., & Bélanger, C. (2015). Emotion regulation and other psychological models for body-focused repetitive behaviors. *Clinical Psychology Review, 33*(6), 745–762. doi:10.1016/j.cpr.2013.05.004. Epub 2013 May 17.

Robertson, M. M. (2012). The Gilles de la Tourette syndrome: The current status. *Archives of Disease in Childhood—Education and Practice, 97*, 166–175.

Seignot, J. N. (1961). [A case of tic of Gilles de la Tourette cured by R 1625.] *Annales de Medecine Psychologique (Paris), 119*(1), 578–579.

Shapiro, A. K. (1970). Gilles de la Tourette's syndrome. Dangers of premature psychologic diagnosis. *New York State Journal of Medicine, 70*(17), 2210–2214.

Shapiro, A. K. (1976). The behavior therapies: Therapeutic breakthrough or latest fad? *American Journal of Psychiatry, 133*(2), 154–159.

Shapiro, A. K., & Shapiro, E. (1968). Treatment of Gilles de la Tourette's Syndrome with haloperidol. *British Journal of Psychiatry, 114*(508), 345–350.

Shapiro, A, K., & Shapiro E. (1971). Clinical dangers of psychological theorizing. The Gilles de la Tourette syndrome. *Psychiatry Quarterly, 45*(2), 159–171.

Shapiro, A. K., Shapiro, E. S., Bruun, R. D., Sweet, R., Wayne, H., & Solomon, G. (1976). Gilles de la Tourette's syndrome: Summary of clinical experience with 250 patients and suggested nomenclature for tic syndromes. *Advances in Neurology, 14*, 277–283.

Shapiro, E. S., Shapiro, A. K., Fulop, G., Hubbard, M., Mandelo, J., Nordlie, J., & Phillips, R. (1989). Controlled study of haloperidol, pimozide, and placebo for the treatment of GTS. *Archives of General Psychiatry, 46*, 722–730.

Shusterman, A., Feld, L., Baer, L., & Keuthen, N. (2009). Affective regulation in trichotillomania: Evidence from a large-scale internet survey. *Behaviour Research and Therapy, 47*, 637–644. doi:10.1016/j.brat.2009.04.004

Spessot, A. L., Plessen, K. J., & Peterson, B. S. (2004). Neuroimaging of developmental psychopathologies: The importance of self-regulatory and neuroplastic processes in adolescence. *Annals of New York Academy of Science, 1021*, 86–104. doi:10.1196/annals.1308.010

Thibault, G. (2009). Électrophysiologie cognitive et motrice du syndrome Gilles de la Tourette. PhD thesis, Université de Montréal, Montréal, Québec.Thibault, G., Felezeu, M., O'Connor, K. P., Todorov, C., Stip, E., & Lavoie, M. E. (2008). Influence of comorbid obsessive-compulsive symptoms on brain event-related potentials in Gilles de la Tourette syndrome. *Progress in Neuro-Psychopharmacology and Biological Psychiatry, 32*, 803–815. doi:10.1016/j.pnpbp.2007.12.016

Thibert, A. L., Day, H. I., & Sandor, P. (1995). Self-concept and self-consciousness in adults with Tourette syndrome. *Canadian Journal of Psychiatry, 40*(1), 35–39.

Thomalla, G., Siebner, H. R., Jonas, M., Baumer, T., Biermann-Ruben, K., Hummel, F., & Munchau, A. (2009). Structural changes in the somatosensory system correlate with tic severity in Gilles de la Tourette syndrome. *Brain, 132*(3), 765–777. doi:10.1093/brain/awn339

Törneke, N. (2010). *Learning RFT: An introduction to relational frame theory and its clinical applications.* Oakland, CA: New Harbinger Publications, Inc.

Verdellen, C., van de Griendt, J., Kriens, S., & van Oostrum, I. (2011). *Tics: Therapist manual.* Amsterdam: Boom Publishers.

Wang, H. S., & Kuo, M. F. (2003). Tourette's syndrome in Taiwan: An epidemiological study of tic disorders in an elementary school at Taipei County. *Brain Development, 25* (Suppl 1), S29–31.

Wile, D. J., & Pringsheim, T. M. (2013). Behavior therapy for Tourette syndrome: A systematic review and meta-analysis. *Current Treatment Options in Neurology, 15*(4), 385–395. doi:10.1007/s11940-013-0238-5

Woods, D. W., & Houghton, D. C. (2015). Evidence-based psychosocial treatments for pediatric body-focused repetitive behavior disorders. *Journal of Clinical Child and Adolescent Psychology, 45*, 227–240. doi:10.1080/15374416.2015.1055860

Woods, D. W., & Marcks, B. A. (2005). Controlled evaluation of an educational intervention used to modify peer attitudes and behavior toward persons with Tourette's syndrome. *Behavior Modification, 29*(6), 900–912. doi:29/6/90010. 1177/0145445505279379

Woods, D. W., & Miltenberger, R. G. (2001). *Tic disorders, trichotillomania, and other repetitive behavior disorders, behavioral approaches to analysis and treatment.* Boston, MA: Kluwer Academic Publishers.

Woods, D. W., Piacentini, J. C., Chang, S. W., Deckersbach, T., Ginsburg, G. S., Peterson, A. L., Scahill, L. D., & Wilhelm, S. (2008). *Managing Tourette syndrome: Therapist guide.* New York: Oxford University Press.

Woods, D. W., Piacentini, J., Himle, M. B., & Chang, S. (2005). Premonitory Urge for Tics Scale (PUTS). *Journal of Developmental and Behavioral Pediatrics, 26*(6), 397–403.

Woods, D. W., Wetterneck, C. T., & Flessner, C. A. (2006). A controlled evaluation of acceptance and commitment therapy plus habit reversal for trichotillomania. *Behavior Research and Therapy, 44*, 639–656.

Wojcieszek, J. M., & Lang, A. E. (1995). Tics. *Movement Disorders, 10*, 2, 224–228.

Author Index

A

Aardema, F.   22, 143
American Psychiatric Association
        10, 12–13, 17
Anderson, M. T.   17
Ascher, E.   9
Azrin, N. H.   17, 19

B

Baer, L.   144
Banerjee, S.   13
Barnes-Holmes, D.   149
Bélanger, C.   143
Berli, K. S.   17
Blanchet P. J.   16, 19
Bloch, M. H.   19
Bohlhalter, S.   15
Bond, F. W.   127–128
Borgeat, F.   16
Borkovec, T. D.   45
Branet, I.   16
Busch, A. M.   19

C

Catrou, J.   9
Cavanna, A. E.   17–18
Cercone J. J.   17
Christenson G. A.   19
Cohen, D. J.   18, 22
Conelea, C. A.   129
Connell, P. H.   10, 14
Corbett, J. A.   10, 14
Crossley, E.   17–18
Crow, S. J.   19

D

Daltroff, W.   9
Dana, C. L.   9
David, K.   17
Davies, W. H.   17
Day, H. I.   18
Day, L.   18
Deckersbach, T.   16
Derby, K. M.   17
Detlor, J.   22
Devilly, G. J.   45

E

Eapen, V.   13

F

Falkenstein, M. J.   19
Fast, D. K.   10
Feld, L.   144
Ferenczi, S.   9
Fine, K. M.   92–93
Flessner, C. A.   19, 31
Forget, J.   13
Freeman, R. D.   10, 13

G

Gagnon, M. M.   19
Gelinas, B. L.   19
Gillanders, D. T.   129–130
Gillberg, C. J.   13
Gilles de la Tourette   14
Golden, G. S.   18
Golomb, R. G.   19
Goris, M.   17

Subject Index

Managing Tic and Habit Disorders: A Cognitive Psychophysiological Approach with Acceptance Strategies, First Edition. Kieron P O'Connor, Marc E Lavoie, and Benjamin Schoendorff.
© 2017 John Wiley & Sons, Ltd. Published 2017 by John Wiley & Sons, Ltd.
Companion Website: www.wiley.com/go/oconnor/managingticandhabitdsorders

Printed and bound by CPI Group (UK) Ltd, Croydon, CR0 4YY

27/10/2024

14580363-0001